'Uterine contractions are felt by many women to sweep towards them, rise in crescendo and then fade away like waves of the sea. . . . A woman must "swim" over the wave and not allow it to envelop her, and to do this she needs to go forward to meet it with her breathing instead of waiting until it is already on her. If she retreats from it it will almost certainly sweep over her. So she sets out to judge its size, and to keep on top of it with her breathing, adapting the rhythm and depth of her breathing to the curve of the wave. As it approaches its crest, her breathing is at its most light and rapid. . . . With each wave of the sea the tide gradually flows farther in, bringing nearer the time when her baby will be in her arms.'

Cover photograph of Hokusai's Wave by courtesy of the British Museum.

Education and Counselling for Childbirth

Sheila Kitzinger

BAILLIÈRE TINDALL · LONDON

A BAILLIÈRE TINDALL book published by
Cassell & Collier Macmillan Publishers Ltd
35 Red Lion Square, London WC1R 4SG
and at Sydney, Auckland, Toronto, Johannesburg
an affiliate of
Macmillan Publishing Co. Inc.
New York

First published 1977

ISBN 0 7020 0642 4 limp

Printed in Great Britain by Cox & Wyman Ltd
London, Fakenham and Reading

In memory of my Mother

Contents

A Note to the Reader

This is not a book about exercises and how to teach them. They are mentioned in passing, but the point of the book is rather different; it is about *the normal life crisis of having a baby*, and how doctors, nurses, midwives, physiotherapists, childbirth educators, psychotherapists and social workers can help a woman, and often the prospective father too, meet the challenge arising from new emotional and social stresses which confront the couple when a baby is on the way. This includes helping the woman towards acquiring techniques for handling her labour so that she has the minimum pain and the maximum confidence, understanding and feeling of well-being. It is very much concerned with how the husband can help his wife and, if he wishes, can share the experience of birth, and how the teacher or counsellor can communicate with him about this.

Because the roots of this book lie in the many hundreds of National Childbirth Trust classes in preparation for childbirth which I have myself taught prospective parents, and countless discussions with them about their feelings throughout the process of pregnancy and birth, I hope that it may also be useful to those men and women who have an opportunity for choice in the childbirth classes they attend, so that they can evaluate what courses have to offer and whether they seem to meet their needs. Up to now many women seeking classes have had to take anything that was available in the area, and there has been some consumer dissatisfaction with classes which involved a few disconnected breathing and relaxation exercises, and a chat over a cup of tea. Now the choice is widening and many expectant mothers have the opportunity to shop around a bit.

From the point of view of those running classes, or giving counsel to childbearing women, too, there are new developments in method and approach, coming from many parts of the world, new techniques for stimulating discussion and for making classes lively groups in which women or couples together can share ideas and find mutual support. Most women who attend classes at present are middle class. Yet they are not the only ones who might benefit from education for birth and parenthood. Perhaps there are other women in our society who need it more, and this might be one way of breaking the cycle of deprivation even before a baby was born into a family, and before the next generation was caught up in it. As an anthropologist, I have had the opportunity of studying women's attitudes to and behaviour in pregnancy and birth in the United States, Latin America, the West Indies and Africa, as well as among immigrant groups in Britain, and have paid particular attention to what is provided for what are often called 'clinic patients'—those who cannot afford to buy medical care—and those mothers who, whether they have money or not, are culturally deprived. So there is a good deal about the underprivileged woman's needs also in these pages.

Ideally, an expectant mother is not really a 'patient' at all. She is not ill and may well be at the peak of health. Her relationship with her doctor during pregnancy is much more one of partnership, and one in which they can make plans together for a safe and happy delivery and in which she can speak frankly about her hopes, fears, and doubts, knowing that she will be heard with sympathetic understanding. Although it may sound easy, this is a task which demands varied skills from the doctor, not the least that of being able to relinquish the social distance and authoritarianism which sometimes marks his relationship with a patient. Moreover, it is not good enough to have all the right *feelings* of friendship towards the woman. He or she must also be able to *communicate* and have appropriate words with which to discuss the enormous changes which are occurring in her body, the emotional adjustments of pregnancy, and the apprehension that is perfectly normal when facing any challenging life crisis. Schools of medicine do not usually teach these skills and obstetricians have to acquire the art the hard way, through experience. Some simply protest that they have no time for it in their busy lives. Nevertheless, although women appreciate a good surgeon when they require one, far more of them welcome the help of an obstetrician who treats them as an equal, gives them a chance to talk, and knows how to offer emotional support.

As nurses and midwives are confronted with more and more machines to operate, some of the skills traditionally associated with midwifery tend to be given less emphasis. There is really no reason why this must be so, for the fact that a fetal monitor is recording every single heartbeat could mean that the midwife might have more, not less, time for her patient and be able to be even more observant of the emotions of labour. In this book I have tried to think what can help not only the midwife who is teaching expectant mothers antenatally but also the one who is concerned to continue giving support and coaching during labour, so that she can carry on the work of the preparation classes. Many women particularly value the presence of another woman who understands what they are feeling, and no machine can ever take the place of a good midwife, both in terms of seeing what is happening—not just to the uterus but to the whole woman—and in giving encouragement and help of the right kind at the right time.

Throughout these pages I am speaking to all the professionals and paraprofessionals involved in maternity care in terms of two roles: those of teacher and counsellor. These roles overlap, of course, but in one way or another every doctor, midwife, social worker and antenatal teacher is both a teacher and a counsellor, and it is important for every worker in this field to be flexible and adapt to the needs of the women they serve and be able to offer teaching, counselling and (most important) *listening* when necessary.

Although I refer to the antenatal teacher as 'she' throughout, more men are getting interested in this work too, and couples are beginning to teach together. This is particularly marked in the United States, but it is happening more and more in Britain also.

I decided to refer to the baby as 'it' in this book. Of course, no baby is. But I knew I would suggest militant feminism if I used 'her' every time. Because I have five daughters myself, it does not come naturally to say 'him' and might also imply that boy babies were the only really important ones. I think that antenatal teachers and others who talk about the baby before it is born may need to do the same, explaining why this is so, or decide to use 'he' and 'she' alternately.

To help women through childbirth is to share a mystery, and a miracle. I remember a Professor of Obstetrics confessing to me that he often had to turn away and surreptitiously wipe his eyes when a baby had been born because he found that he was sharing the parents' delight and tears of joy were streaming down his own cheeks. It is also to touch life at a key point in the social system, when generation gives way to generation, when bitterness and frustration and a sense of worthlessness can be handed down to the next generation, or the opportunity taken to grow in understanding and love. There is more to having a baby than simply pushing an occipito-anterior out into the world. Birth is also implicitly an assent to life. Those who help women in childbirth have the privilege of sharing that act of assent.

Standlake Manor   SHEILA KITZINGER
Oxfordshire
January 1977

Acknowledgements

This book owes a great deal to the many antenatal teaching students I have taught both as a tutor of the National Childbirth Trust and lecturing abroad in the United States, Canada, Bogota, Israel and South Africa. I always learn more than I teach and find that every workshop I have taught has been for me an enriching experience.

I also want to thank my colleagues with whom I have discussed projects and problems, especially the Advanced Teachers of the NCT, prenatal teachers with the International Childbirth Education Association, the American Society for Psychoprophylaxis in Obstetrics and the Paramedical Association for Childbirth Education in Johannesburg, members of the International Society for Psychosomatic Medicine in Obstetrics and Gynaecology, my own Study Group on Home Confinements, and many other obstetricians, midwives, physiotherapists, psychiatrists, paediatricians and general practitioners who have made helpful suggestions, and have given me food for thought and modified my ideas and practice—especially Professor Peter Huntingford, Professor Norman Morris, Mrs Bianca Gordon, Dr Martin Richards and Dr Aidan Macfarlane. To single out any of my colleagues whom I feel have most deeply influenced the formation of my own views is, perhaps, invidious. But I cannot omit thanking in particular: Mrs Gwen Rankin, Mrs Charity Torrance, Mrs Joan Gibson, Mrs Betty Parsons, Mrs Margaret Williams, Mrs Elizabeth Bing in New York, Dr Ruth Wilf in Philadelphia, Mrs Margot Edward in California and Mrs Norma Swenson of the Boston Women's Health Book Collective.

I owe an enormous debt to Mrs Audrey Macefield, my secretary, whose sharp eye, unfailing good humour and concentrated hard work actually got the book written.

The kernels of some of the chapters in this book were articles published in journals and magazines, and I am grateful to the following in particular for allowing me to use material derived from articles I wrote for them: *New Society, Mother & Baby, Mother, Forum, Vogue, The Journal of the Marriage Guidance Council, Midwife & Health Visitor, Nursing Mirror,* the *Newsletter of the Obstetric Association of Chartered Physiotherapists,* the *Journal of the Institute of Group Psychoanalysis, CIBA Review, The Practitioner, British Journal of Sexual Medicine, General Practitioner,* and the *Teachers' Broadsheet of the National Childbirth Trust.*

Working towards Childbirth

I

The Teacher

Antenatal teaching is a new profession demanding new and varied skills. It is not teaching women physical jerks, or labour drills or even 'relaxation classes', but educating for childbirth and parenthood. Such a wider approach inevitably makes the role of those who guide women through this period a more complex and difficult task and also a much more challenging and rewarding one than, perhaps, we have thought of it before.

Many short courses intended for midwives, health visitors or physiotherapists and run by their professional bodies are designed to top up information and to provide a forum for discussion. These are by no means the only categories of women who can provide a skilled source of antenatal teachers and counsellors.

Organizations concerned with childbirth education have sprung up all over the world and include the International Childbirth Education Association; the American Society for Psychoprophylaxis in Obstetrics; the Paramedical Association for Childbirth Education in South Africa; and in Australia and New Zealand, the Childbirth Education Association and the National Childbirth Trust of Australia and the Federation of New Zealand Parents Centres Incorporated respectively.

In Britain the National Childbirth Trust,* for example, trains women from many different backgrounds over a period of one or two years in the theory of childbirth education, conducting classes

* 9 Queensborough Terrace, Bayswater, London W2.

and group discussions, and in counselling. This is done by means of a tutorial system combined with a series of one- two- and three-day seminars and study days. When possible the student is put in contact with a local group of teachers who discuss problems together and share ideas. Selection procedures are designed to encourage those with potential skills and the right sort of personality, and at the same time discourage those who see this teaching merely as a solution to their *own* problems—of loneliness, frustration, or an unhappy marriage perhaps—and those who have a doctrinaire approach. Neither physiotherapists nor midwives are considered by the NCT to be fully equipped to do antenatal teaching without further study, practice and exploration of different approaches.

In the United States the International Childbirth Education Association (ICEA)* selects on the basis of applicants' professional and personal experience of family-centred maternity care and their answers to questions such as: Why do you feel that childbirth education is important? Why do you want to teach it? What skills do you have that will aid in teaching? What books have you read relating to childbirth and breast feeding? Many ICEA groups have two interviews with an intending teacher, a first in which they get to know her as a person and learn about what she sees as the primary goals of classes. If she is accepted for teacher training she observes classes, after which there is another interview, at which a student's abilities are assessed.

The physiotherapist's knowledge of body mechanics and the experience of conducting labours which the midwife acquires are both important in childbirth education. But they are not sufficient to make a good antenatal teacher. Psychological and social factors are intricately intertwined with physiological ones in the experience of childbearing and in the process of labour. Those who have skills in psychology and sociology may therefore be in an equally good initial position from which to work towards that combination of skills indispensable for really effective antenatal teaching. (Indeed the way things are, psychological and sociological techniques may be rather more difficult to acquire on top of physiological knowledge than physiology is for those who have been trained in the social and

* 14423 S.E. 23rd Pl. Bellevue, Washington D.C. 98007.

psychological fields.) In addition, nothing can replace the experience of having oneself joyfully born one's own babies in full awareness, and of having had to face and cope with some of the psychological and social problems which confront most women in childbearing and child rearing. But simply having given birth happily oneself is inadequate as a basis for good teaching. Too often then a woman has a very one-sided picture of labour, and merely superimposes on other women ideals of how labour ought to be.

Labour is a highly personal experience, and every woman has a right to her *own* experience and to be honest about the emotions she feels. Joy tends to be catching, and when a teacher has enjoyed her own births this is valuable because she infuses her own sense of wonder and keen pleasure into her relations with those she teaches. But she must go on from there, learn how difficult labour can be for some women, and develop an understanding of all the stresses that may be involved.

No one can hope to start training in antenatal teaching with all these different qualifications already combined. But even where, for example, the personal experience is lacking, a dedicated midwife or psychologist—or even, given the personal experience, someone who has learnt how to absorb different scientific disciplines and is prepared to wade through the heavy obstetric textbooks and the diffuse psychological literature bearing on these issues—can train herself to the point where she will perhaps at times make mistakes (in what profession does that never occur?) but where the good she does will far outweigh the cases that lead to disappointment, and where she can thus be of real service to other women. To some extent experience can be handed down, and aspiring antenatal teachers have much to learn from those with years of experience behind them, can sit in on their classes and participate in seminar discussions with others converging on this new subject from other points of departure. In the last resort as in other branches of education and psychology, there is no substitute for practice. An antenatal teacher has never finished training. Certainly after sixteen years I for one feel it is a bad week when I do not learn something new that I wish I had been able to use before.

Apart from knowledge and experience, teaching makes its special demands of personality. The quality of the human relationship between teacher and taught may be difficult to measure, but it is this, rather than the subject taught or the teaching techniques employed, which is the essence of education. In antenatal teaching, the teacher–pupil relationship is all the more complicated since the delicate adjustment of the childbearing woman to her own body through the different months of pregnancy and in the different phases of the extraordinary activity of labour, and to her family, the future baby, and a new pattern of family relationships, involves her in constant psychological change and development throughout pregnancy—changes which will obviously affect and change her relationship with the teacher.

A useful exercise for any antenatal teacher is to discuss with a group of colleagues what one is aiming at in teaching. I see the aim of education for birth neither as achieving childbirth *without* something—pain, fear, or whatever, nor, indeed, even *with* something—that special miracle ingredient Sz XL99—dignity, triumph, or conscious control. Having a baby may involve all these things, but the introduction of such concepts can suggest either that pain or apprehension are somehow unworthy and are not to be acknowledged by any self-respecting woman or that there is some particular attribute or skill which makes childbirth a marvellous experience, and without it the less said the better!

There is no such thing as success or failure in childbirth; there is simply a woman having a baby. The essence of her experience is not merely that of labouring, although birth often involves extremely hard work (harder work than a woman has ever in her life known before) but of *giving*, of opening herself up physically and emotionally. She is not enacting a performance. She is surrendering herself to a new and revealing experience and offering her body in the creation of a new life. This giving is really a sort of loving not so much of the baby—because he or she is still a fantasy child—but it involves acceptance of her own body and, in particular, a glad acceptance of the vagina as an organ which can open and give birth. It also means that she must be able to accept her own emotions, the light and the dark ones, the positive and the negative. The art of giving birth comes to some by happy accident, to some by concentrated study, thought and practice, to some because they can utterly trust and rely on someone —the doctor or midwife perhaps—and to others again by inexplicable grace.

A woman's body opens up, and the apparently impossible, the almost incomprehensible, turns into reality and achievement. Just as a crocus pushes through the cracks in the garden paving—tender, fragile, soft, vulnerable but with the relentless power of life sweeping through it—a woman *gives* birth. It is the capacity to give which childbirth education can foster. This giving is a matter not only of giving birth but of being able to give in the marriage, and in the relationship with the baby and the growing child.

The teacher is working not only with a woman who presents herself at classes nor even with a couple but the couple in their relationships with all the other people—professional helpers, family members and others—who are involved in the birth of that baby.

The manner in which antenatal teachers see themselves profoundly affects how they teach and what they have to offer. The information at their disposal, their teaching techniques, the quality of their voices, the skill they exhibit in their demonstrations and lectures are all secondary to this self-perception.

When conducting seminars and study days with antenatal teachers in Britain and in the United States, I often suggest that they explore the ways in which we see our roles as teachers and also the way we see that our students perceive us.

Teachers see themselves above all as 'friendly and emotionally supportive', 'compassionate and caring', 'with a warm personality', and 'interested in me [the student] as a person'. They also perceive themselves as 'enthusiastic' or even 'overenthusiastic'—one problem being that they feel that a midwife or doctor might be left 'to pick up the shattered illusions'. They are problem-solving, ready to listen, and 'delight in answering questions', although they sometimes get confused or find themselves unable to come up with an answer. Some evidently feel that they are standing on a knife edge between being supportive to their students' needs, including awareness of their fears and anxieties, and feeling that there is danger in this and 'not wanting to be too emotionally involved'. They see the class atmosphere as friendly, relaxed, informal and happy. 'Free and easy' 'not a bit clinical', and 'home from home' are expressions some teachers use. They stress their own striving to be 'truthful', that they 'answer questions honestly' and 'tell us about all the things that can go wrong and how to cope with them'. 'She will find out things she doesn't know' and 'admits to not knowing all the answers'. Sincerity is obviously considered an important quality, as is readiness to admit gaps in information.

There are some marked differences between the American and British teachers in their attitudes to themselves. These cross-cultural differences in role perception are apparent, not only in the teacher's goals or even of her image of herself in relation to the students but in the relation between the teacher and students and medical profession. The British teachers often see themselves as being 'quiet and diffident', 'shy', 'hesitant'. The teachers, we are told, 'find it hard to push themselves', do not have a 'strong enough personality', 'lack confidence', and also face problems in verbal expression amounting even to being 'inarticulate at times'. The single fact that emerges above all others is that the British teachers are torn between perception of themselves as self-confident and assured in style, which they see as important in teaching, and as completely lacking in confidence.

The American teachers tend to speak about themselves with greater confidence and with overt aggression towards obstetricians. They are particularly resistant to what they see as the seductive friendliness of the obstetrician who seems to be saying, 'Little woman, depend on me. Do not bother your pretty head about these matters. You can trust me!' One wonders whether some male obstetricians are filling a father role just as the midwife in Britain is often cast, in spite of her own wishes, into the role of a good or bad mother.

We need to know more about the perception of obstetricians and midwives by the patient, her husband *and* the antenatal teacher before we can gain any understanding of their interrelationships and their ability to work effectively as members of a team. This needs to be done when teachers meet together to discuss their problems.

It is a subject we cannot afford to shelve, to some extent because the expectant mother is an unusual kind of patient. Traditionally the role of the patient is that of someone who is ill, and therefore dependent, handicapped and socially deviant. The feelings of alienation felt by many women about the maternity care they are receiving is in part a product of this role which is superimposed on them at a time when they are in a state of health and well-being. When women visited the local doctor's surgery and had their babies with a midwife at home they were not cast in the sick role with anything like the enforced passivity and virtual immobility of the hospital patient who is linked to an intravenous drip and wired to a fetal monitor.

We are faced with a challenge in the health services. The role of prospective parents needs to be redefined if we are to avoid ambiguity and confusion in the relations between maternity patients and the medical personnel advising and caring for them. This is a social task of some magnitude, involving education of doctors and nurses as well as patients, so that all their expectations are appropriate and interaction can be reciprocal.

The atmosphere of a class is set more by the teacher than by the physical surroundings. Antenatal teachers sometimes tend to skate over the surface of experiences which are for most women deep and precious and to concern themselves with the physical and measurable. Too many still do not know enough about the psychological differences and emotional problems of the mothers in our care and teach as if all the women had to do was to obey the rules and then their labours 'should' bring satisfaction and a feeling of triumph. But we know that this is not the case. The woman who has all the tricks of technique, has practised assiduously, and follows this up with a perfectly straightforward, apparently easy labour may be just the one who feels a tremendous discontent and dissatisfaction afterwards and feels in some indefinable way that she has failed. Whereas the woman who has been bad at relaxing, seems keyed up, perhaps has a difficult labour, may come through it radiant and thrilled to bits with herself, her husband and the baby.

A woman once came to me who had had three lessons a week from the fourth month of her first pregnancy in a European country, had been the 'star' of the class and showed me the most elaborate breathing and other exercises she had learned to perform there.

She could pant abdominally so that her abdominal wall shook like a belly dancer's! But her labour was disastrous. 'I was an utter flop,' she explained, 'and my teacher had thought I was so marvellous!' The second birth was approached with anxiety, her confidence now shattered, and she attended the hospital's antenatal classes in England, where they concentrated on body mechanics for pregnancy, on slow deep breathing and elementary relaxation. This was nearly as bad as the first experience. Neither teacher had really known her as a person. Each had concentrated on techniques.

'Trust' in doctor or midwife, valuable as it is, is not always a sure recipe for a happy labour. It may be enough for a woman to be healthy and hopeful and to know what is happening to her; it may be enough for her to be looking forward to her baby and to trust her attendants; enough for her to learn some breathing exercises and leave it at that. But it may not. Time and time again I meet women who need more time and care than is given by an overworked general practitioner or the enthusiastic but psychologically un-informed antenatal teacher—women who need an opportunity to talk, express their fears and worries, and work through their problems in pregnancy in readiness for the responsibilities of motherhood. As one severely depressed woman said: 'I am so full that I could burst with tears. I want so much to speak myself out.'

Preparation for childbirth must take account of the differences between women and their varying needs, and as a teacher you should at least allow time for your pupils to talk—talk together with one another and talk privately with you if they want to.

The teacher's task in this is never to impose judgement, never to criticize, never to rush in with snap solutions, however obvious they may seem to be. You are not there as a mother substitute, a drill sergeant, or a conjuror who, with a Hey presto! displays the sleight of hand and can make all problems vanish; nor to poke around shining a powerful light in the mental dustbins, weasling out guilty secrets. You are there to draw out each individual's capacity for arriving at an awareness of and sensitive response to her body and the voluntary activity required of her during labour. You are there to get to know your pupils by talking through their problems with them and, too, to help build up in them a confidence in their ability not only to bear a child but to be a good mother. It is easy for a teacher to fall into the trap of seeing the main function as one of reassurance. This is not true emotional support and often entails the dismissal of unpleasant facts and a turning away from reality. 'I should just forget that. Put it behind you. Don't dwell on such thoughts. I'm sure everything will be all right. You've got to think of the future' . . . or 'your child' . . . or 'your husband'. The support which is worthwhile can accept reality and looks it square in the face. This involves knowing when and how to mirror stress.

Part of our function is to act as a looking-glass to some of the doubts and fears which the pupil presents and not to rush in with the answer or to correct her. There are points at which one has to wait and simply reflect back what one has been given, to hold a watching brief and to tolerate the pupil's anxiety. The teacher who has a great social conscience, who goes round purging the pupils' minds and filling them with good positive things, cannot tolerate anxiety. We can only work at the necessary level if we can tolerate inaction.

In all this we must remember that in everything we do and say we must help each woman to relate herself more closely and in greater understanding to her husband, and must do and say nothing which could detract from the value of the relationship which they may be only just starting out on together. A woman's relationship with the teacher is ephemeral and transitory; one hopes her marriage will be permanent.

This awareness of childbirth as part of a woman's whole psycho-sexual life—not simply as an isolated occurrence at one end of her body—must not only permeate all the teaching and affect the verbal imagery used and the way in which it is put over but should involve sensitivity to difficulties that a woman may be confronting in her marriage, in the way she sees herself as a woman, in her attitudes to motherhood, even in her relations with her own parents. Married teachers who have children themselves ought to have a tremendous advantage over anyone else, but some of them undervalue their own experience of living and are reticent about just the things that expectant mothers most want to discuss.

Teachers rarely need to give advice; in fact, it is usually better if they do not, and those who are most enthusiastic about proffering advice are usually the last ones who should be giving it. The teacher should be prepared to listen and wait patiently. From each woman you will learn *something* if you have ears to hear.

2

The Interview

'The idea of interviewing and counselling terrifies me,' said a teaching colleague. 'The very words scare me.' This is a pity, for at its simplest the interview is a conversation in which you get the chance to know a person better. Counselling may or may not be a part of it, but in the interview with an expectant mother, where the interviewer wants to give emotional support, it is a natural ingredient. Counselling can take place both with individuals and with groups and is interwoven with teaching throughout the course of antenatal classes. It need not be directive and best achieves its purpose when it enables people to sort things out for themselves.

On the other hand, the interview with a pregnant woman is more than a friendly chat; it is initiated for a specific purpose and focused on the pregnancy and birth. It is as well for you as the interviewer to state the purpose as you see it, so that both members of the partnership—and this is what it should be, however short it is—know what sort of communication is relevant. To put it another way, let us say that the *content area* is explicitly stated. The doctor, midwife, social worker or antenatal teacher will be looking for different things in their interviews, but whatever the content area, two basic attitudes are important: *a live interest* in knowing the person and *openness* to what she offers.★

When wanting to get answers to questions and tapping people for

★ See Allen J. Elenow and Scott N. Swischer, *Interviewing and Patient Care* (New York, O.U.P., 1972).

information, whether or not this involves a written questionnaire, there is a risk that you will be interested only in the answers given to questions which you consider are really relevant to the task in hand, and all else is considered waste material. In a true conversation each subject of discussion arises quite naturally out of something that has gone before, and there is a flow from one topic to another. This is how it is with a good interview; that is, its shape results from developing themes—a shape which belongs uniquely to that interview and to no other. In this it is essential to remember that the respondent provides the material of the interview, not the questioner.

When I started interviewing in anthropological field work many years ago, my supervisor at Oxford gave me some advice: 'Squeeze them as you would a lemon.' (Brutal as this sounds, he was not a bit this sort of man, and was completely incapable of treating any other human being in this way.) His advice provided a valuable stimulus, and made me think what I was really trying to do in an interview. For there is a great deal more to a lemon than its juice: flesh, rind, pips, taste, colour, perfume and zest. You cannot accurately describe a lemon simply in terms of its juice, any more than you can accurately describe a person by the answers he or she gives to a list of questions, however exhaustive. Even when not 'loaded', the form of the question, and the series of questions, in itself dictates the kind of response one obtains.

Moreover, the interviewer is an inherent part of the interview and affects what happens during it. However little they know about each other beforehand and whether they are socially separate, even though physically close, because of their widely disparate social statuses (demonstrated visually, for instance, by a white coat), interviewer and interviewed are involved in a relationship which is going on all the time, even when they are not talking.

The antenatal teacher who is concerned with the interview not only to get information but as an integral part of a helping relationship might introduce the interview by saying: 'I think it is a good idea for us to meet like this so that I can learn about you as a person, and you have an opportunity to discuss anything which may be on your mind, and ask questions about classes, and so on.'

More is being done in the interview than getting material, however important the content of the interview. The relationship created is always more significant than the data collected. One aim of every interviewer should be that the respondent goes away thinking 'I enjoyed that!' Yet the interview *process*—the developing interaction between the participants—is important because it is part of this relationship and because it profoundly affects the quality and range of information acquired. So you can help yourself by exploring the ways in which you interact with the person being interviewed.

The interview process is largely a product of the way in which both participants see their interacting roles. Here some models of different kinds of doctor/patient relationships may be able to clarify the scene: There are three kinds of interaction which occur as the result of culturally defined doctor/patient roles. They are called Activity–Passivity, Guidance–Cooperation and Mutual Participation.*

In the first, the doctor is authoritarian and the patient is completely dependent, tries to please, and takes no active role in treatment. When the Queen inspects a row of guardsmen she initiates any conversation, asking questions which the soldier answers briefly. We should be very surprised if the guardsman turned to Her Majesty and asked How are the corgies? or Where do you plan to go for your holiday?

In Guidance–Cooperation, the patient has a greater sense of self-direction, but the doctor maintains authoritarian status, deciding the way the interview should go, the information required, and the area to be investigated, and sometimes misses important things because of this.

In the Mutual Participation relationship, both members actively join together to explore the subject of the interview, and the patient also takes responsibility for its outcome. This interaction we can call a *symmetrical relationship*. Quite apart from what is learned in the interview, such a relationship can have a therapeutic function, as the participant is no longer helpless and passive but able to assess her

* M. H. Hollander and T. S. Szasz, *The Psychology of Medical Practice* (Philadelphia, Saunders, 1958).

part and to plan and organize action in the future; this in itself reduces anxiety.

The model for the interview between teacher or counsellor and the expectant mother should be that of the symmetrical relationship between social equals—one of mutual participation. To offer anything less is to miss a valuable opportunity for understanding, and for building together a basis on which to work towards birth and parenthood.

A person-to-person relationship involves an exchange, and the more fully we can make the initial interview situation an exchange of attention, interest and information—the more completely reciprocal the relationship can be, that is—the firmer the basis is on which teaching or counselling can be built in subsequent encounters. Stefan Zweig goes so far as to say that

The act of interviewing . . . can be a graceful and joyful act, enjoyed by the two sides and suffered by neither. What is more, my contention is that unless it becomes such an act, it will only fail in its main function. One cannot conduct an interview by bombarding one's victim with a barrage of questions, which is only tiresome and tiring for both sides. The only way is to make an interview an enjoyable social act, both for the interviewer and the respondent, a two-way traffic, so that the respondent feels not a 'victim' but a true partner, a true conversationalist.*

In practice this means that you approach respondents not with I want you to learn or even Can I help you? but with the attitude: Can you help me understand?

Some respondents are obviously more informative than others. Sometimes you get a stream of communication and there is hardly time to make note of it all. Sometimes the informant seems to have her mind on other things. You must expect to like certain women more than others, and they in their turn will sometimes like you and sometimes be distrustful or suspicious. Be honest about your own emotions and make a note of them when the interview is written up, which should always be as soon as possible after it has been terminated. Thus space must always be left between interviews for this important writing-up. If using a tape recorder, however, for which

* Stefan Zweig, *In Quest of Fellowship* (London, Heinemann, 1965).

you must get each woman's permission, you can use the time of the interview to record visual and other aspects of it, leaving the tape to do the auditory recording.

The questions asked can either be highly specific, requiring only Yes or No answers or short factual responses, or they can be open-ended. The open-ended kind are far more effective at getting the person interviewed to talk, and to think, and also in allowing the interviewer deeper insight. The most effective questions are those which provide a broad opening to a topic of such a type that the respondent has to think before she can answer.

The interviewer also needs to be a facilitator, that is, you open the door to the expression of attitudes and ideas and discussion of topics which might previously have been closed. There are countless ways of giving encouragement in this, one of the most obvious of which is a nod. The use of 'Um . . . um-um' is also useful.

At the University of Oregon Medical School forty men were given interviews lasting three-quarters of an hour. In the second quarter of an hour period of twenty of these interviews the researcher said 'Um-um . . .' at intervals. As a result, the respondents increased their talking time from a mean of thirty-seven seconds in the first period of the interview to forty-eight seconds in the second period—an increase of 31 per cent. The interviewer stopped saying 'Um-um . . .' in the last quarter hour, and the average length of talking went back to thirty-nine seconds. With a control group of twenty, the interviewer gave no verbal reinforcement at all, and they never changed their average length of speech, talking for a mean of thirty seconds in the first quarter of an hour, thirty in the second and twenty-eight seconds in the third period.★ Other verbal expressions, such as 'Yes', 'I see', 'I don't quite get that', 'I don't think I really understand', or 'I'm not clear why you are asking this. Can you tell me a bit more about that?' can also facilitate communication. Sometimes just a questioning look or even a movement towards the respondent will encourage her to go on.

Occasionally put what the respondent has said into your own words to check that you have not misunderstood, or draw forth further clarification of the subject. This has to be carefully and

★ Materozzo *et al.*, *Psychotherapy*, Vol. 1, No. 3 (1965).

sympathetically done or she may feel dismissed, the whole subject put in a nutshell as if it were not worthy of the importance she attached to it. Also avoid trite generalizations which make her feel she is being put into a category rather than approached as an individual.

The use of what has been called *confrontation* is also valid in some situations: 'I notice you look anxious'; 'I get the impression that you are extremely angry about that'; 'You seem very happy about this'; 'This seems to make you miserable'; 'I get the feeling that you do not find this easy to talk about'. You describe what you see in the respondent's behaviour or appearance. When this is sympathetically done it shows that the interviewer is picking up not only what is said but the mood in which it is said. We are saying, in effect, 'I notice what you are telling me, and I understand'. It is much better for you, the interviewer, to describe your responses to the person being interviewed in this way than to attack her with direct questions such as: Why are you so quiet? Why are you biting your nails? or Do you realize that you are tense? Questions such as these find no place in a sympathetic interview (they are much more the sort of questions that angry parents put to their children with whom they are annoyed, and since they invite evasion, falsehood and self-justification, they are not such a good idea then either!).

Confrontation, although it may sound aggressive, is not really so. It is a means by which the respondent is helped to face reality, or what appears to be the interviewer to be reality, given the information at her disposal. In facing the reality, and possibly anxiety-laden issues, it is not so much forcing someone else to come up against the unpleasant or inevitable as *standing beside* the other person and looking at the problem or the challenge *together*. Use sympathetic confrontation when verbal and nonverbal behaviour are unsynchronized when, for example, she says: 'I am not afraid about having a baby,' but acts as if she were anxious, twisting her legs, screwing up a handkerchief in her fingers, and furrowing her brow. She may not be anxious about birth, but if you point out to her, with sensitivity and care, that you noticed that she is sitting right on the edge of her chair and is clenching her fist and biting her lip, she may stop, be aware of her own actions for the first time, and then say: 'Yes, well,

I suppose I am worried really. But it isn't having the baby. It is about afterwards. I just feel I haven't any maternal instincts', or something of this kind.

The interviewer must also make it clear to the respondent that she is *accepted*. Probably most people are not as confident or self-assured as they seem, and a good many are obviously nervous and apprehensive. The interviewer can say, 'Yes, I see', 'I understand', 'I know', or 'I can imagine how you feel' at appropriate points in the conversation, and thus affirm the identity of the other, and her right to the ideas and feelings she has. Especially when strong emotions have been expressed can support of this kind be valuable, because often the respondent wonders if she has made a fool of herself in giving way to her feelings.

If the person interviewed is finding it really difficult to express herself it may help to simply repeat her last phrase with an upward inflection. For example, suppose she says 'I feel depressed', and then seems to dry up, one might gently ask Depressed? Occasionally slightly raised eyebrows are sufficient in themselves. This is a technique which can be overused and become merely mechanical unless it is employed with sensitivity, but it is one which can often get an interview out of a rut.

When working with a notebook, avoid writing at the point when the informant is obviously expressing something which she finds difficult to put into words, or when she is trying to say something that is embarrassingly intimate for her. This is not necessarily anything to do with sex; in some cultures anything to do with money proves even more embarrassing, and one can easily discover a good deal about people's sex lives but very little about their financial state. To stop writing is an indication that you are not hungrily fixing on just these subjects which are hardest for the informant to talk about and allows you to leave your face available and open. When interviews take this turn it may be important for the respondent to be able to see your facial expression easily, to see sympathy, understanding and acceptance on your face, and to be in relation with you as a person and not merely as a note-taker. Sometimes the situation is such that you can look straight at the respondent and she at you. Sometimes, when tension is greater, you will find that you quite spontaneously gaze away from her and offer, as it were, a stillness in which her words can be received and pondered. The basis of all this is that you are not automatically recording and doing the work a tape recorder could do anyway but are involved in a *helping relationship*.

The interview consists of pauses as well as talking, and time may have to be given for reflective silences. It is easy when one first starts interviewing to go at it like a bull at a gate, and out of your eagerness and concern to do it well, coupled with anxiety that you are not competent, to fire questions at the person with such rapidity that the attacked individual raises defences against investigation. A good interviewer is a good *listener*. You should be able to sit in a relaxed and comfortable way, opening yourself to the other person with interest, acceptance and attentiveness. This entails being able to tolerate silence. 'The most common reason clinicians interrupt silences is their own tension'.★

Never be afraid of silence, when working either with individuals or with groups. Simply sit and wait. If you are not concerned to tap informants as fast and as hard as you can there is time for spaces in discussion, and these can be much more valuable than rushing on to the next question. Sometimes the comments that arise following a period of silence in a relaxed atmosphere, the half-expressed thoughts, the introduction of a query, the recounting of a dream or something that somebody said that has been on her mind, can lead to much deeper perceptiveness on the part of the interviewer.

The capacity to sit still on stage without becoming tense or making nervous movements is one of the first skills of an actor. To be able to sit and listen is the first skill of an interviewer. To listen with obvious interest is psychologically supportive, even if the interviewer has nothing else to offer. When a person becomes distressed or gives way to the expression of any disturbing emotion, the interviewer should let her cry or be angry, and wait, without interrupting or rushing in with soothing words of reassurance. Emotional support should be given only *after* such emotions have had opportunity of free expression. The interviewer's task is not to dam up emotion but to allow it to be expressed within a safe context.

★ Elenow and Swischer, *Interviewing and Patient Care*.

The 'stillness' provides a clue to the essence of any interview which is designed to be not only informative but, if required, supportive and therapeutic. And for the interviewer, like an actor, it starts with the ability to sit quite still, without jiggling with pencils or paper-clips or showing any nervous mannerisms which obtrude on the interview. One must, in fact, be able to tolerate not only silence when necessary but also inaction, both at the level of physical still-ness, and emotionally, in terms of being able to avoid giving advice.

Much of what can be learned in the interview comes not from words but from nonverbal behaviour. Part of the task of a good interviewer, whether it is somebody obtaining a case history or a psychotherapist listening to a patient recounting his problems, is to become aware of the pattern of muscular tensions which affect intonation, respiration, physical movements, posture and gait. A detailed interview cannot be written simply in terms of what a person said. You will find, in fact, that you have to develop a sort of personal shorthand to describe these phenomena—the point at which the person being interviewed drops her voice for instance or when her words seem to rush out in a spate of enthusiasm or when she moves her chair slightly farther away or smiles or frowns. To the person starting this sort of work for the first time this may seem a counsel of perfection, but interviewing is really not just a craft but an art, and gradually the interviewer will acquire new observational skills and new techniques of exploring ideas and attitudes together, so that the interview then becomes something which not only pro-vides you with more and more detailed information, but involves an essentially satisfying relationship which gives pleasure to both parti-cipants.

The Interview with Husband and Wife

Some of the potential of the interview is demonstrated in what can be done in the private (and strictly confidential) consultation, in a peaceful, relaxed atmosphere, with husband and wife together, held normally at the start of a course of classes (just before or soon after) and repeated when there is special need, for example if the woman is encountering any grave emotional problem, such as depression, at intervals through the later weeks of pregnancy, and postnatally if required. This consultation lasts for a minimum of one hour, and sometimes considerably longer. The usual pattern is for each couple to have one private consultation before they start lessons. If there is a long gap of more than a few weeks between the end of the course and the expected date of delivery you may be able to offer a second private consultation during that period. With the last 100 women I have taught, 96 have had a joint consultation with their husbands, the remainder being those whose husbands were abroad or unavoidably absent for other reasons (and then the women had interviews alone). It is noticeable that it is after this interview that the husband who is concerned about his wife in late pregnancy will ring me, rather than expecting the wife to ring if she is distressed, and that we become from the interview on much more a 'working team'. All personal details are obtained at the first interview, and I aim to get some idea of her state of mind and her feelings about the pregnancy. With multigravidae it is useful to get full details of previous pregnancies and labours and the woman's subjective experience of them.

The first objection to such an interview is that it is time-consuming, and this cannot be denied. There is an argument, however, for having one or two fewer classes in the course if this presents the opportunity of setting aside a day, or several evenings, for this private interviewing. In this interview the teacher sets the scene for the husband's participation in the antenatal preparation and the labour and helps the couple to make it a shared experience.

Having a baby used to be a matter for the woman, with her mother standing in the background giving advice and information, and often the folklore, including the old wives' tales, which did so much harm. Nowadays it is much more something for husband and wife to share together. There are still some men who express their insecurity by saying that they do not want to get involved in women's things, and who feel their manliness is being challenged. But the majority of those coming to classes approach childbirth with curiosity and interest and, apart from wondering whether they are going to make fools of themselves playing an unfamiliar role and an understandable nervousness that it involves unpleasant procedures, want to help their wives and to give them the practical assistance and emotional support which can contribute towards a never-to-be forgotten experience when they together bring their baby into the world.

Some men think that it is 'good form' to hand their wives over into the care of experts and retire from the scene. They feel that the professional must have so much more knowledge than they can possibly have that they will be in the way and that they have no function in the labour room. The antenatal teacher should explain to these men that hospital staff are usually extremely busy and involved with more than one patient at a time, and can rarely give the constant companionship and uninterrupted loving care which a woman often craves as she is swept through the unfamiliar physical and emotional experiences of labour. She needs her man with her—not simply as an onlooker but as someone who has studied what childbirth involves and what her antenatal preparation has been.

It is a good idea to see both prospective parents, even when they are unmarried, and when they are not planning on continuing their relationship. The man who merely acknowledges paternity is often diffident and ashamed about getting further involved. If necessary ring him up and explain how he can help you to help her in this way. He nearly always comes. Even if a man has nothing else to offer a woman he can give her emotional support, and this especially if there seems little point in them marrying. It is bound to be painful for them both if they decide to part with the baby, but this can be an important experience for them and help them to grow in understanding. There is nothing to be gained from pretending that these experiences do not hurt, or that it is something which they quickly put behind them. But inherent in the crisis is a challenge, and one which may in the end, in spite of the distress it brings, be integrated into their lives, separately or together, as a constructive experience.

The first meeting the teacher has with a couple is, as we have seen, an occasion to explore what the birth and the coming baby means for them and any particular problems they may be facing. As the teacher notes the couples' name, address, and the expected date of delivery the man is summing up the teacher and beginning to relax. The spotlight is off him. A point is soon reached when the woman turns to him and asks his opinion. The teacher may ask about menstruation, for instance, and enquire whether her periods were regular, what they were like, and whether she had any premenstrual tension or pain during the period. Occasionally a man will offer information and a discussion starts from this topic. Or it may be in answer to a question as to whether the baby was planned or not, and they may start to say something about their sense of indecision, or discussion they had about wanting a baby. It may be in response to the question, What sort of time did your mother have when she had her babies? The woman may say, 'Oh, she never talks about things like that', and the husband makes an amused and perhaps derogatory comment. She replies to him and they explain that subjects concerned with sex have always been taboo, and he explains what effect he feels this has had on his wife's upbringing and character. Obviously the questions you as the teacher ask are directly related to what has gone before, for you are not firing items from a questionnaire at them, but engaged in a conversation.

One effect of our teaching is frequently to change our pupil's sense of the clean and the unclean. In all human societies there are values relating to this area of the sacred on the one hand and the profane on the other, the holy and the ordinary day-to-day, the tabooed or unclean and the clean. When we are discussing attitudes to the body I always try to find out amongst my pupils those who suffer from constipation, because it helps me to know their attitude to the excretory processes. It is customary in antenatal teaching to make a bridge between sensations of defecation and those experienced during the second stage of labour, but it is important to bear in mind that women who find defecation disturbing carry these feelings over into childbirth, and that the analogy may be an entirely unsuitable one for them.

Let us take just four couples whom I have not selected for their interest or peculiarity but who happened to be in one course of classes. (I have made alterations in the material so that they are not identifiable.)

I asked Anna, for example, how she was feeling about the pregnancy, because she had told me that the first four months were miserable, and her husband replied, 'She was very upset all last evening'. Anna explained that she was depressed, and added, 'You get to the point where you can't sleep any more'. A question as to how a woman is sleeping is important because an initial plea for help is often expressed in the form of a statement that she cannot sleep. In this case a discussion ensued between husband and wife about her emotional reactions, in which the teacher was just an onlooker. The husband was a musician, and Anna turned to me and said, 'His music drives me up the wall'. He was bewildered, and there was some risk that in offering sympathy to Anna he would be alienated and feel that the two women were combining against him. I listened for a while, and then said to Anna, 'Tell me some of the things he's good at!' She replied, 'He is very good with cats. If he treats me like he treats the cats, that's fine!' It was from here that we were able to discuss her feelings of being unloved and rejected, both emotionally and physically as it turned out, during the pregnancy, which they had not been able to talk about directly with each other before.

Linette and Charles were not married. They had met at a psychiatric clinic after he had failed his finals, and were both on drugs. She was still severely depressed. At first she did not speak at all, and Charles answered the factual questions. I asked, 'How are you sleeping?' and she started to talk hesitantly and to tell me how unhappy she was. This was their first meeting for four weeks, because Charles had decided that they should go their separate ways, and he had only turned up now because I had asked expressly that he should attend if possible and said it would be a help to me if he would come. I asked, 'How are you feeling now?' 'Alone . . . isolated', she replied. Charles obviously felt uncomfortable and wanted to raise this conversation to a philosophical plane. 'A dialectic is going on inside her!' he exclaimed, and then he confronted me. 'We are living our own way of life, trying to find proper morals beyond any social institutions.' I nodded and said 'I understand'. 'I am torn between the way Charles sees morality and my parents' desires for me,' she said. 'They think "*my* husband", "*my* child".' 'A thoroughly dishonest approach!', Charles added. I asked how she was living now and where she was getting money from. Charles said that her parents were paying for her support. I did not comment, and there was a short silence. A little later I asked, 'Why did you start a baby?' and she replied, 'I thought it was . . . time.' 'It didn't just happen,' he insisted. At the time I felt I could have been of little help to this couple, but two things certainly emerged from it: Charles attended classes with Linette, and at the next class he told me he had been able to get an overdraft to support her financially. Perhaps we should note in passing that it is not the function of the interview to pass judgement in any way on a couple, and a teacher whose own life style is very different from the man and woman whom she is meeting has to be careful to avoid judgement.

Sophia and her husband were a very different couple. He was an obstetrician. Here again, it was when I asked how Sophia was sleeping that she told me she was 'terribly full of thoughts' and kept having nightmares, including a repeated one of a jumbo jet 'sinking out of the sky' and all life in it being obliterated. It struck me that her own body was the 'jumbo jet' and that she was a very frightened woman. This was their second baby. The first birth had been a disastrous experience in which the husband had been invited by the doctor doing the delivery to assist, and he said, 'The only way I know how to deal with a pregnant lady is the doctor's way'. He said he saw now that it was as if he had attacked her. They had separated afterwards, had sought marriage guidance and now were determined to make a success of their marriage and the second birth. They were both highly motivated to making good use of the interview, and discussion was easy. One main function of the interview from my point of view was that I had been given clear indication that in order to give emotional support to Sophia I should approach him as a husband and father and not in his threatening role as an obstetrician.

When I asked Linda if she had 'any worries about having the baby', she replied that she was not so much concerned about the birth, but wondered 'how I am going to cope after, looking after this new baby', and it was at this point that George told me how much *he* was looking forward to parenthood: 'I feel like doing everything, changing the nappies and everything. I am so excited.' It became clear that Linda had been required to act the part of a radiant expectant mother, both by George and by her Greek parents-in-law, who were delighted at the coming birth of what they were quite sure must be a grandson. Since Linda was not even sure that she could provide them with the sex they desired she was left feeling a reproductive failure and someone who did not matter for herself but only for her maternal functions in relation to George's family. They both needed an opportunity to discuss this together, and the interview provided such an occasion.

The interview with the couple does not end with talking. An important aspect of my approach to counselling is that we go on from there to do work with body awareness, and the second part of the initial private consultation is spent in learning Touch Relaxation, that is, the couple engage in a task together and focus on practical preparation for birth. The joint activity involves concentrated attention by the husband in helping his wife and it means that they leave the interview with a commitment to practise together. This is an important factor in the marriage, because it is easy for each to shelve responsibility on to the other if action is left for the future only and if support is purely verbal at this stage. Good intentions can easily be expressed in words, and then forgotten.

So there comes a point in the interview when the teacher says, 'I'm going to show you something that I should like you to start working on together now', and they leave with a defined task.

Marriage Counselling in Pregnancy

Not all teachers will feel that they should attempt counselling, but it is because antenatal teachers are working with bodies, and not only talking with couples, that they have a tool at their disposal which few marriage counsellors possess. Words do not always provide solutions. Frequently they delay flexible adaptation in response to stress. Confrontation, explanation, justification, and the discussion that was fully intended to be quiet, reasonable and understanding, all too often turn out to create a worse mess, with recrimination, accusation, and further confusion and hate. Sometimes we need to by-pass words.

I have found that the sort of relaxation involved in antenatal preparation is also relevant not only for meeting the inevitable stresses of everyday life but for facilitating a constructively adaptive response to marriage problems. The very fact that both face a physical rather than a purely verbal task, and one in which they share, forms part of the therapy.

If relaxation is to be useful in this context, it must not become simply a discipline that is *imposed* on one partner by the other: 'Relax, relax', 'I *am* relaxed!' Rather, it must be genuinely shared and should form part of the continuing nonverbal language that exists anyway between people who live in proximity, particularly if the relationship is basically one of love.

For many people relaxation is a solitary activity, when they lie on the floor and go limp and try to imagine they are floating on a cloud or attempt to 'think of nothing'. The approach which I suggest is one involving the couple together, and, far from being solitary, is part of a dialogue: that is, it is a form of communication.

Where there is sexual dysfunction or there are problems in relating to each other physically, the study of relaxation together—involving close physical contact, but in the absence of an imposed erotic goal —can lead to an intensified awareness of each other's needs, and often to increased sensual delight. This is the major theme of Masters and Johnson's work on sexual dysfunction: that goal-oriented sexual exercises lead to a sense of urgency and concern about likely failure, which introduces further disharmony and in-coordination; couples need time in which they feel they are not being pushed to perform.* Exploring sensation and creating new body-awareness through relaxation is an approach to coping with these problems which allows pleasure on the way towards a possible solution, and is not simply concentrated on the need to find a solution.

Masters and Johnson stressed that sex was natural, and not something that had to be learned. But to be able to enjoy it, it may be necessary to remove barriers. These barriers are for the most part those of contracted musculature which prevents psychophysical coordination, necessary for the performance of any smooth, rhythmic process, whether this be playing the piano, driving a car, walk-

* William H. Masters and Virginia E. Johnson, *Human Sexual Response* (Boston, Little, Brown, 1966); *Human Sexual Inadequacy* (Edinburgh, Churchill, 1970).

ing and running, digestion, defecation, giving birth, or making love.

Part of the task is to discover what causes tension, exactly how each reacts to stress, which parts of the body contract giving a stimulus, and how this makes one *feel*. So there must also be time for discussion about what is happening and why, and of what each becomes aware of in the other.

In Chapter 11 I discuss techniques of teaching relaxation, with reference to the work of Jacobson, adapted Method acting exercises, and using the approach of Touch Relaxation.

NOTES AND RECORDS

The Teacher's Case Records

Although it may seem a counsel of perfection, the larger the classes the more need is there for you to keep records which can supplement your memory. If groups are large you can try to arrange time before each when you can sit down with the records and check up on women's names and other material. After each class you should plan into your schedule another space when you can write up anything relevant.

These records can get very dog-eared unless they are kept on firm cards which can be stapled together when necessary. This is a format I have found useful:

Name: Address: Telephone No: E.D.D.   Previous
                                              Employment:
                                              (underline if
                                              continued in
                                              pregnancy)

Where to be delivered.   Doctor.   Details of previous labours and her subjective experience of them.
Note on general health and on health during pregnancy.
Ask 'How are you sleeping?' Note reply.
(Inability to sleep may be evidence of anxiety.)
Information on her expressed goals regarding prenatal preparation; stimulated by questions such as 'Why would you like to come to classes?' 'What do you want to learn?' 'What do you think will help?'

Note on her own mother's, and perhaps sister's, experiences of birth. Ask 'What sort of time did she have?' Do you know anything about what happened when she had her first child? Has she said anything about it?' Note if she sees these relatives much. Note any traumatic experiences among friends or neighbours, discussion of which may arise spontaneously out of these queries.

In a joint husband–wife interview much more can be obtained, and is discussed further in Chapters 6 and 16.

Affix any notes from doctor. Note any communication of information to doctors concerned and add to this card other information obtained during teaching course. Finally affix the labour report.

The Log Book of Labour

For this an ordinary school notebook is suitable. I always suggest that the expectant mother uses the first half of this for notes of things she wants to remember from classes, and for writing any queries she may have for the class teacher or for her doctor or midwife. (This is important, as she may forget when actually confronted by them.)

For the labour log book itself, double pages are conveniently divided into columns, with a margin at one side in which the time is noted.

Column 1. Observed signs of labour and its progress, written up by the mother and/or father.

Column 2. Techniques of adjustment used by mother at this phase, written up by father and/or mother.

Column 3. The assistance and/or medication given at this phase of labour by staff.

When such a record is written up in full with the actions and comments of various members of the labour team much can be learned from each account.

Notes after Classes

After at least some sessions you will help yourself to become more receptive to what your pupils have to offer if you write up exactly what happened, or those parts of it you were observant enough to notice, between members of the group in their relations with each other, and between each pupil and yourself. A special book or file kept for these notes will form a record of what can be virtually a journey of discovery for the teacher.

3

Group Dynamics

There is no one 'right' way to work with groups. Although I personally prefer working with small groups of not more than about sixteen members at most, and find groups of twelve people probably the easiest to work with, some classes, especially those in hospitals, simply have to be large, although even there it may be possible to break up the large class into smaller groups.

Historically, antenatal teaching grew out of physiotherapy and remedial gymnastics on the one hand, and the class for midwifery instruction, held in a lecture theatre, with the speaker segregated behind a table or lectern with her notes, on the other. These origins are still clearly visible in the way in which many classes are run, with separate sessions for exercises and for instruction, often conducted by different teachers, the one being all action, sometimes accompanied by barrack-square commands of a kind which seem little to do with having a baby, and the other being entirely static, the pupils sitting drinking in the information which is being handed out to them. In neither of these is there any true 'group process', since relationships between participants are minimal, and the class looks to the teacher to keep it running.

There are classes I have seen conducted in East Germany, with the expectant mothers sitting round a large table, a white-coated instructor up one end, and pictures of Pavlov and Marx looking down with what must surely be astonishment from the walls, while intricate drawings of female anatomy are constructed on the blackboard. Occasionally the instructor pauses, asks 'Any questions?' and when there are none, says 'Oh, good. Let us continue then'. In France there are classes where pupils sit assiduously writing notes for all the world as if they had to pass their *baccalaureat* in childbirth. And there are those in other countries of Europe where a sort of elephant ballet of pregnant women is conducted. All these methods work, I am sure, because they involve concentrated care of the mother and a concentration of attention on her part, both essential factors in preparation. But they all miss out on the advantages which can be gained from using the group to help itself and stimulating women to support and learn from each other and share experiences.

These authoritarian and didactic methods of lecture theatre and physical education class in antenatal teaching derive from a simplistic psychology which reduces education to the level of a series of conditioned reflexes. At the other extreme is the soothing chat about labour, which is intended to reassure, but which assumes that expectant mothers are not very bright and circumvents their real problems and feelings.

The Nature of the Group

In a workshop conducted in South Africa at the invitation of the Paramedical Association for Childbirth Education, I suggested that we try to sort out the differences between an audience and a school class and a squad. The physiotherapists, occupational therapists and midwives taking part came up with some carefully thought out conclusions, all relevant to the classes we are running, to the nature of the relationships between teacher and taught, and to those between members of the class. We decided that a squad was an active, disciplined and often highly trained unit in which the participants' role was to obey and conform. One main characteristic of the squad was that it was drilled and regimented. It was the most rigidly organized unit under consideration. An audience had a largely anonymous membership; that is, members did not usually know each other, and there was little interaction between them as individuals. They listened to what was being communicated to them, without being seen themselves, except as an amorphous mass. Although not passive, they were usually required to be receiving for the most part, and it was the actors or musicians who did most of the giving. (It is in reaction to this relatively passive role that many theatre groups are trying to engage their audiences in more positive and creative interaction with them.) In a class the pupils have come to learn, or are supposed to have come to learn, a frequently predefined task, although teachers and taught do not necessarily have a common purpose. One person is in authority and has responsibility to instruct the class members, among whom there may be some interaction, often disapproved of, and some active participation. (Here again, many teachers are reacting against the idea of the class as primarily a training group and against the minimal interaction between teacher and taught and between class members themselves, associated with authoritarian teaching.)

We then considered how the antenatal group which we aimed to create differed from a squad, an audience and a school class. It was agreed that members should, above all, have a feeling of belonging and that there should be interaction with the teacher and with each other. They shared common goals, which were not imposed from outside, or by the teacher, but which resulted from their similar interests and needs and which she helped them to define. It was the teacher's responsibility to discover the needs of her group and respond to them. She should be able to manipulate activity in the group without dominating it, and to stimulate and draw out ideas and feelings, so that everyone was motivated to participate fully. Her function was partly that of a teacher, but primarily that of a facilitator. Let us examine how in practice these goals can be sought with a group of expectant mothers.

I might have called this chapter Group Leadership or Group Counselling, but I chose the word *dynamics* because I wanted to make clear my conviction that the best teaching can be done when the teacher does not 'hold the floor' all the time, but is an active member of the group, sharing experiences with the other members; is not 'out in front of' the group, confronting it with information, but has the skill and confidence to be able to stand back sometimes and let the members explore subjects themselves; and encourages discussion in such a way that any member feels free to introduce a subject which is on her mind, whether or not it is in the syllabus.

The mutual support which then emerges in the group of women who are all passing through a similar experience is vitally important, and is probably more significant than any relationship with pupils which the teacher establishes as a fact-giver, clarifier or adviser. One function is to be a 'bridge' over which members of the group can communicate with each other, and in this respect to help them put into words ideas they may find difficulty in expressing. This involves the knowledge of when to become submerged in the group, and to let it act, itself a difficult art to acquire, especially for the extrovert or overtalkative teacher.

The nucleus of what I attempt to do in classes can be summed up in two words: *discussion* and *participation*. Of course I instruct, explain, teach adaptive techniques for labour, and check relaxation and breathing, but threaded through this there is an interchange of ideas between all members of the group. They take the suggestions and look them over and test them in terms of their own experience and the real world in which they live. All information has much more relevance to each member's own life when they can do this, and when new facts and new aspects of the childbearing experience can be related to those they already know.

The beginner antenatal teacher is often concerned that discussion may get out of hand. To this I would say:

When discussion starts, be grateful, even if it may seem irrelevant and does not fit into the syllabus you had so carefully planned. Use every opportunity for building up group feeling, and let the syllabus slide if spontaneous discussion develops at any point in a class. You may find they are ready for information you intended to give at the next or subsequent class. If so, it is not they who are wrong but the syllabus which is at fault. They are ripe for the information *then*, at that moment; change the syllabus and give them what they are asking for.

Good teachers will probably find that discussion spontaneously develops in each class, often towards the end in 'young' groups, and they ask appropriate questions to stimulate further thinking and to help the expression of fears, apprehensions, doubts. If necessary they protect any member of the group who seems the odd one out and whose experience of life somehow runs counter to that of other members.

Direct questions from the teacher to the group can stimulate discussion, but it is essential to be ready to follow up a question with another, which perhaps puts the same query in a different way, or with subsidiary questions. In this way group members are encouraged to think about subjects which they may not see as directly relevant to classes, but which raise important topics connected with adjustment to birth and parenthood.

Questions should never be fired at a group in rapid succession. Two clusters of questions—a leading or main theme one and a group of subsidiary questions—are ample for any class. Group members then take over the discussion, asking questions themselves, and not only of the teacher but of the group in general. When group dynamics are good, members focus on each other no less than on the teacher.

Often when a question is asked by one member it is right not to answer it, but to turn to the group and ask What do *you* think? The teacher can learn a great deal in this way. This method of working with groups is no concession, something you as teacher do simply as a manoeuvre designed to reassure, but provides essential information and is something you cannot afford to be without.

The wording of questions which the teacher introduces in the group depends on the nature of the class, the socioeconomic and educational levels of its members, and above all on what has gone before. Queries need not be questions at all, but statements with an upward inflection of the voice, or they may be prefaced by phrases such as: I wonder whether, or I'd be interested to hear whether you think that. . . . What the teacher is doing is to make links between areas of experience with which most group members may have seen no, or slight, connection. They may be practising relaxation assiduously for labour, for instance, and you ask, 'Do you think this relaxation may be useful after the baby comes at all?' You might go on from there to suggest, 'Let's think of the future and foresee some of the situations when relaxation may help. Perhaps those of you who already have babies can advise us here?' . . . and so on.

Following on the same theme, the teacher might ask an individual, 'How did you feel when you brought Angela [or whatever the baby's name is] home from hospital and realized that she was your total responsibility?' Obviously if you already know your students through a private interview, you are in a much better position to ask this of someone who can describe vividly the loneliness, fear and anxiety which many new mothers experience. Perhaps you turn to another member and ask, 'Can you remember how you felt at first when you were alone in the house and the baby cried?' This might lead on to a discussion with multiparae about the different confused and conflicting feelings parents may have when their babies cry, and what they do about these feelings. This is a discussion which goes best when new parents come back to a class to tell about their labours and what it is like to have a new baby in the house, as the experience is immediate for them.

If the visits from new parents are arranged at the end of classes occasionally, the theme of a discussion merges with the meeting with the new parents. They will have heard about the birth and how they coped, and the teacher can then say, 'We've been discussing the emotions a new baby can arouse in the parents. Can you tell us how you felt?' They will describe positive as well as negative emotions, which is what is needed. This may be one of the best ways in which to help parents most at risk of violence towards a baby, to realize even before the child is born some of the emotional conflicts involved in new parenthood, to tolerate these disturbing feelings, and to know how to handle them.

The teacher could have linked the question about the postpartum period with other aspects of relaxation in everyday life. 'Jane, you plan to go back to work after a while. Think of being in the office. Is there anything which often makes you tense up there? Can you tell us about it?' and then, perhaps, 'Which of us are car drivers? Let's think about getting tense when driving' ... 'Suppose you aren't going out to work like Jane, and you are stuck at home with the washing up and two dozen dirty nappies? ... Have any of you who have had a baby experienced that? Tell us about it, will you? What did you find yourself doing?' It is important not to let discussion about neuromuscular tension get bogged down with words. It should always be related to actually working with bodies. This is where the Stanislavsky approach described on pages 154–6 may be helpful. The teacher picks up a vital point and says, 'We can probably all imagine just how that feels, can't we?' and then builds a bridge between the area of tension that has been described and a similar, but not necessarily identical, experience everyone in the group has had.

A woman who has not had her baby cannot know what it is like to be isolated and trapped in an empty house with a screaming infant and dirt, faeces and other mess to clear up. But everyone can discuss what it is to be 'trapped'. 'Has anyone here ever been physically trapped, perhaps in a cupboard or a lift? Can you tell me how you felt? Did you tense up? Did it affect your breathing, do you think?' and the like. (I remember as a child getting stuck in a large underground drainpipe which we used to think it great fun to explore, and may introduce this anecdote to stimulate discussion.)

If participants are slow to express ideas, anecdotes can be used as a stimulus for the group: I used to know a girl who felt ... *or* I remember when I had my first baby. ... In discussion on subjects concerning which there may be a special sensitivity or reluctance to talk, the group leader must avoid direct questioning or the exposure of any one member of the group. One can ask, for example, 'What do you think women worry most about during pregnancy?' or of women from a different culture about whose ideas you may have little firsthand knowledge, 'Have you heard of any things that women do, or are careful not to do, so that they make a healthy baby?' That is, one is careful not to suggest This is what *you* believe; this is *your* erroneous idea. Discussion will soon turn to personal attitudes, thoughts and fears, even if these are carefully wrapped up as My sister used to ... or My neighbour says. ...

Because this is real, and not spurious, information that the teacher is requesting, she will need to keep note of suggestions made by the mothers themselves, of the relevance or ineffectiveness of images she used and of techniques taught for labour, noting not only verbal but nonverbal behaviour which provides clues to this. We have already seen that this can teach us a good deal about a woman's expectations of labour and what can be done to assist her, and developing out of this, help us understand something of her body concept and of the total picture of physical well-being and wholeness on the one hand and of sickness and accident on the other.

Antenatal Teaching and Psychotherapy

Some antenatal teachers shy away from the whole idea of psychotherapy, because they feel they are likely to get into deep waters if they attempt to use a skill for which they were not trained, and often because they suspect that it involves 'meddling' with the unconscious, recalling forgotten childhood trauma and uncovering secrets which are best left buried. Psychotherapy in the context of antenatal teaching quite simply means that one is 'helping the mind' and, in some cases, because by interacting with others the group members can become more aware of themselves and better able to come to terms with 'inner needs and the demands of outer reality',★ is able to share in a process of emotional healing.

I suppose there are few antenatal teachers who would say, as I heard one affirm defensively some years ago, 'All my girls are normal!' Even those who believe that all the women coming to them are 'normal' would hardly assert that they are all happy. To do so would be to ignore the fact that many expectant mothers are beset by fears, not necessarily about the birth but perhaps about their ability to cope as mothers, their marriages, or their personalities or even the capacity for coherent thinking, which they feel are being eroded. The very fact of being pregnant raises new questions and poses problems.

Whether or not we feel comfortable with it, antenatal teaching is work which has psychotherapeutic potential. We can either do it with our eyes closed, or can discover some of the implications of our words and actions. The trouble is that the teachers who deny any psychotherapeutic possibilities in what they are doing are the very ones who may be doing harm, because they are unaware of the effect of the relationship with their pupils and of their response to them.

★ S. H. Foulkes and E. J. Anthony, *Group Psychotherapy* (London, Penguin, 1965).

Psychotherapy in the antenatal group, whether with expectant mothers only or with couples together (and I think that increasingly we shall find more and more couples wanting to share their preparation), does not involve any digging down into the unconscious or a forced invasion of privacy. It is very much in the 'here and now', and its focus is on the members' capacity to respond to the stresses inherent in pregnancy, to prepare for the birth emotionally as well as physically, and to gain understanding of some of the changes that occur with parenthood.

The Group as a Transitional Ritual

The antenatal class provides for expectant mothers something corresponding to the transitional rituals, or *rites de passage*, between two significant points of the life cycle—that of being a bride and that of being a mother—which exist in peasant and primitive societies. We sometimes act as if in our highly evolved industrial society we did not need such rituals, as if we could take childbearing in our stride, and that it is enough to learn the manual and organizational techniques which the next stage of life requires of us. Preparation for parenthood is not just a technical matter—learning how to change a nappy or bath a newborn baby, for example. It is concerned with our intimate feelings about ourselves as we adjust to new social roles.

In most primitive and some advanced societies groups are formed for warriors, or boys or girls at puberty, or of old men or old women, who are at the same stage of life, face the same problems, and have similar tasks. In them they get companionship and mutual support, and learn the ways in which things are done in their society, are inculcated with the values of the group, and initiated into the responsibilities which confront and the dangers which threaten them. Nothing quite like this exists for expectant mothers—who are passing through a period of immense change, both physiologically and emotionally.

Pregnancy can also provide the extra stress that accentuates marriage problems—the woman who wants to shut her husband out from her life, the man who is jealous of the unborn child in the same way as he was of a younger sibling, the woman who leans on her mother, or the one who suffers from feelings of inferiority because she really resents her femininity—for all these pregnancy can be a threat to the marriage. The group in preparation for childbirth fulfils a vital need and becomes a *rite de passage* from one state of social identity to another.

The Group as Peer Support System

When we face problems in life it is easy to forget that there are others confronting the same difficulties and worries, whether these are associated with work, illness, bereavement, marriage, children's behaviour or the life crisis of having a baby. It is strange, perhaps, how often people believe that *their* problems are unique. One of the first things that the new antenatal teacher discovers is the sense of relief which pregnant women often express when they start to talk about things that are on their minds and find that many of the other women feel exactly the same way. When people at the same phase of their lives, or encountering disturbance in their accustomed patterns of living, reach out to share thoughts and feelings and to help each other, we have a valuable means of community self-help which we can call *peer group support*. In a highly fragmentized industrial society these people often do not meet each other in the normal course of events, and they struggle on without the support which is there if only they knew how to find it. So from one point of view, although the expectant mother initially seeks the tools, of information, and breathing and relaxation techniques, which she needs to equip her for a specific task, an antenatal class is also a way in which expectant mothers, who are together passing through the experience of pregnancy and facing the challenge of birth, form a supporting peer group with which to explore the emotional aspects of childbearing.

We have seen how in the group members have the opportunity to share vicariously the experience of birth as others have their babies, and then come to tell at firsthand about their labours, the difficulties they may have faced, and the ways in which they coped and were helped. This vicarious experience of living through childbirth and responding to challenge, combined with discussion about maternal emotions, the effect of the new baby on the marriage, and about how the woman sees her social role adapted to changed circumstances, are all important ways in which members of the peer group can support each other.

Touching

Antenatal teaching is not just a matter of talking. Because it is anticipated that we shall be working with and through *bodies* ante-natal teachers have techniques at their disposal which the psycho-therapist and the marriage counsellor may not possess. Important among these is *touch*, a nonverbal tactile language which can be used both for communication of feeling and to help a person relax and to relate better to her own body. Thus it is expected that we shall do massage. In a class consisting of women only this is usually prac-tised with women working together in pairs, while in the class con-sisting of couples the husbands learn how to do Touch Relaxation with their wives. I suggest to the group that this touch can be used in a very positive way if the woman being massaged relaxes *towards* the touching hands, and that then it becomes something in which she actively participates, rather than a passive process.★

The use of touch in this way has obvious psychosexual connota-tions, and when couples are relaxed and comfortable, discussion often quite naturally turns to changes in the marriage, to feelings about personal psychosexual functioning, and to the basic trust or distrust which a person feels about his or her own body.

For many members of the group, talking probably does not seem the point of meeting together, but nevertheless discussion grows spontaneously out of physical movements and exercises for breath-ing and relaxation. It is probably less strained and deliberate, and less circumscribed by notions of what we *ought* to be talking about, or the socially correct attitudes, because of this. The words and ideas which find expression are a by-product of activity and, as such, are

★ The method of Touch Relaxation is described in detail on pages 156–61, and also in my book *The Experience of Childbirth*, 4th ed. (London, Penguin, 1974).

rarely examined in terms of standards which ought to be expressed or values which one is bound to defend.

Labour: A Social Situation

Exploration of the roles of doctor, patient, husband and midwife, and occasionally the use of psychodrama, can help women to anticipate labour not only as a predominantly physiological or even as an individual emotional process but as an exercise in human relations. It is this for which so many women are ill-prepared in the modern hospital. Doctors, midwives, labouring women and their husbands and mothers and mothers-in-law, all have emotional lives of their own, and interact with each other through the stresses of pregnancy and the drama of birth.

If a nurse is present in the group, for instance, and also a woman who approaches midwives as authority figures with whom she has an infantile and dependent relationship, or one of open revolt and hostility—reenacting highly charged situations of her own childhood in her relationship with the 'midwife–mother'—we may act a scene from labour. It is, perhaps, at the late first stage, or pain period, of a long and rather difficult labour in which the woman is under great stress, that I suggest that the real nurse act the part of the mother, and the mother who is overdependent on or hostile to midwives act the part of the midwife. Encouraged to express whatever they feel when locked in this drama, they begin to understand what is involved for the others, and something of their own comprehension of the often intense emotions with which a woman claims the right—or feels herself unable to claim it—to replace her own mother and to take her place with a baby of her own.

Birth is not only the end of a pregnancy but the beginning of parenthood. It is not simply a grand *finale*, but opens a door onto a new life experience and new social functions. In the classes couples hear at firsthand many descriptions of labour (not a single one of which may be according to the textbook), actually handle new babies, and quickly come to realize that birth and motherhood can be subjectively experienced as very different things for each woman and involve widely varying perceptions of the self. They see that there is no one 'right' way to have a baby, and also that there is a wide range of emotions that the new mother may experience which have nothing to do with what they previously thought of as 'maternal instincts' or with the tenderness which one anticipates feeling about a small baby, but which involves rage, guilt, jealousy, frustration, and even hatred of the newborn. Postpartum support is also a natural extension of the work of the group. Women often maintain contact with each other after childbirth, couples meet each other, baby-sit for each other, and go out together, and informal subgroups are formed which support each other during the early months of parenthood. The special ways in which childbirth education groups can give support during this fourth trimester of pregnancy are described in Chapter 21.

In the groups the use of vivid stimuli, in the form of audio-visual aids, discussed more fully in Chapter 4, can also trigger off discussion. A tennis ball pressed through a sock, with a small hole cut in the heel for the anus, and another large one in the toe end for the vagina, can stimulate discussion about feelings of pressure and fullness behind the rectum and anus, associated responses in defecation, and concepts of dirt and cleanliness in relation to body functions. A doll being pressed through a foam rubber vagina stimulates discussion about sensations of distension on the perineum, and feelings of being 'too small down there'—a recurrent theme in the body image of middle-class English women. One of these teaching aids produces its own psychodrama, the tape-recording of one of my own labours.

When all members of the group understand the basic techniques designed to assist adjustment to uterine contractions they enact the posture and movements, the respiratory patterns and the other neuro-muscular responses appropriate to the birth situation while listening for their 'cues' to one of these tape-recordings. As the newborn child tumbles into the world crying loudly, as the parents are heard laughing with joy, and then go on to describe the baby and to talk together with love, it is obviously an emotional experience for all members of the group, and one in which they achieve identification with the labouring woman. They can thus anticipate some of the positive emotions which can be so powerful in childbirth if they are given a chance of expression. They have acquired a 'set' towards a certain capacity for feeling which may be inhibited in the woman who is merely processed through antenatal clinic and labour ward, and in whom feeling may be denied in order to have a quiet, obedient and passive patient.

The Life Cycle of a Group

Groups, like people, have lives of their own. They have an infancy, youth, maturity and old age, and one can expect different things of them at the changing phases of their lives. Because this is so, you as teacher adapt yourself, use different stimuli and prompting, and can find you are filling a different role *vis-à-vis* the group, at these varying phases. Characteristically with the very new group the members look to you as a leader and parent or authority figure for guidance and may feel slightly uncomfortable if you explain that you do not see your role in this way; they have hardly looked at each other yet, and in the very first class one of your responsibilities is to help them to relate to each other, to approach each other as friends, to learn something about each other and find out what they have in common (even if it is only, at first, their names and when they expect their babies), and to discover ways in which they can provide mutual support. When discussion first starts in a newly formed group the members are rather apprehensive, though curious, and tend to look to the teacher for consent, but this should not persist if the group develops a life of its own, and if you know when to fade into the background and be content to observe, when to be silent, and when to say just the few words that will help forward their relationships one with the other. You need to learn how to stand by to control without dominating, and how to draw out the person who needs encouragement, to suggest, for example, that one woman has a particularly useful bit of experience that would be of value to the rest.

In the newborn group people are often anxious and wonder what they have 'let themselves in for', and it is easy for the teacher to underestimate this anxiety. I remember one woman coming to a class held in my own home, in a comfortable room with flowers, pictures and soft lighting, and I was so much out of tune with what she was experiencing that I was amazed when she said to me as she left, 'I'm so glad that's over now! I actually enjoyed it. But it was like coming to the dentist!' I understood more what a very nervous father-to-be was going through when he came in with his arms stiff by his body, shoulders hunched up, and a pipe clenched in his teeth. He was a rather passive participant, but as he got up to go he turned to me and said, 'Thank heaven! Now I see what it's all about. But I wondered what you were going to do to me!' His wife explained, 'He didn't want to come because he thought he would have to lie down and you were going to massage him!' It shows that he must have relaxed that when I said, 'Ah, that's for *next* time!' he went off laughing, *and* turned up for the next class!

When the teacher can help the members of a new group start to discover their common problems and goals they immediately find it easier to talk, and the group starts functioning. A simple way of doing this is to divide the group in pairs, asking people not to select anyone whom they knew before, and give them two or three minutes for first one to find out about the other, and then for the respondent in the first conversation to be the main questioner in the second. If couples are taking part in the class, I introduce two men to each other, and find that this quickly puts husbands at their ease. Each person then tells the group about the person with whom he or she has been talking. We always use first names at all classes, and this includes my own first name, of course.

A phenomenon which occurs again and again with new groups is one which is sometimes called the *mirror phenomenon*. As discussion gets under way each member gets reflected, as in a mirror, an image of himself or herself in the other members of the group. The most obvious way in which this occurs in the antenatal class is that each woman is eyeing the other expectant mothers to see if they are more or less pregnant, and whether they show their pregnancies more or less. This is one of the first subjects which comes up in discussion, sometimes with slightly embarrassed apologies that one is not so far advanced in pregnancy as another member. Members respond with evident pleasure when they discover they are having babies with the same obstetrician or midwife, in the same hospital, or at the same time, or that they went to the same school, or both have husbands in similar occupations, or two-year-old toddlers. They seem to be looking into the group eager to get an image of themselves returned in this way; this concerns not only facts such as these but attitudes and feelings. When these start to find expression in discussion, and especially when even subjects which are painful or embarrassing can be discussed, the group has really taken off and has a momentum of its own.

Another phenomenon which always occurs is that of role-playing. Group members spontaneously cast themselves, and are cast by the other members, into familiar roles. There is usually one who remembers things that the others forget, and acts as the memory for the group. There may be one who acts the part of the scapegoat, who is always late, can never do the exercises and get the breathing wrong. There is an exhibitionist, and a masochist who recounts tales of terrible labours, and obviously is enjoying all the discomforts of pregnancy. There is one who expresses a sense of independence and adventure. Then there is the fighter, who may be the same person. The fighter is going to take on her doctor single-handed and tell him that she is going to have her baby *her* way. Most groups have a conciliator who is concerned to make the peace between group members, and between the fighters and adventurers and the outside society. Almost always there is a doubter, who raises the awkward questions and is never completely convinced—a very healthy situation to have in any group! There may be a 'little girl' who acts the part of naïveté and innocence, to whom everyone else has to explain things, and who is the group's baby! One person usually assumes the role of the mother to the group; she may be a grand multipara and speaks with the voice of experience and wisdom.

The function of the teacher is not to prevent these characters from emerging, but rather to help them to see how they all, to some extent, share these qualities, and that there is in all of us a 'mother', a 'baby', a 'fighter', and so on. The teacher may turn to the group and ask, 'Do any of you feel like this too?' If the teacher can do this, group members start to learn from each other in a way which is enriching, over and above any facts about labour they may acquire from the classes, or any techniques they may learn for handling contractions.

But a word of warning here: this is not intended as a method of manipulating a situation in which the uncontrolled expression of emotions is given free rein, or in which people are encouraged to expose themselves in a way of which they may be ashamed afterwards.

Sensitivity and Encounter Groups

The goals of the antenatal classes are quite different from those of sensitivity or encounter groups. The teacher accepts the responsibility of accompanying and guiding the group members through the changes of pregnancy and birth. This sense of responsibility is important, and is noticeably absent in some sensitivity training. A famous sensitivity leader was once asked what he would do if a member of his encounter group committed suicide after it was finished, and he replied that this was nothing to do with him. People must be free agents. One critic of this approach, says that 'We must consider encounter groups in the same way that we consider other experimentation with human subjects.'* He contrasts the role of the sensitivity trainer with that of the psychoanalyst and comments that

traditionally, the practitioner, the companion through the process of change, assumed a special responsibility to guide the person into this new status and to help him through any unforeseen consequences. In encounter groups, however, the responsibility ends with the final session.

So whatever emotions are going to be expressed in the antenatal group are the teacher's continuing responsibility, which she can never abrogate. You should always remember that however well you have taught a class, and whatever has happened in it which you, or the members, found stimulating and exciting, you bear some responsibility, too, for what happens to the pregnant woman when she leaves the class and goes home, and the effects of what has occurred in the class on her relationship with her husband, her doctor and midwife, and perhaps also with other members of her family.

* Kurt Back, *Beyond Words: The Story of Sensitivity Training and the Encounter Movement* (New York, Russell Sage Foundation, 1972).

As an antenatal teacher you need to sharpen your awareness of what is happening around you in the relations between people and in the hints you can get from their words and actions of processes taking place in their inner lives. At the same time you can gradually build up the ability to analyse what is taking place in the group, to be aware of the stresses and strains between members, and the ways in which they 'use' each other.

The range of roles enacted is not haphazard. In any fairly mixed group there are women who will relate to others in the group as mothers, or older or younger sisters, so that one also gets a playing out of relationships in the family. Where there are nurses, social workers or teachers, one may get a similar acting out of the emotions the woman feels towards nurses, teachers or social workers, and these in their turn may express attitudes they have towards other women who are their patients, pupils or clients.

The ability to observe what is happening in a group is gradually acquired, and does not spring up full-fledged after reading a book about it. It helps to have someone else who is experienced with analysing sit in on classes and to be able to spend time discussing with him or her afterwards exactly what happened, and the personalities and interrelationships of the members. At first one is so concerned to teach effectively that it is asking almost too much to observe minutely at the same time.

Start observations with very simple obvious behaviour and record such things as who chooses to sit next to whom and where friendships, or antipathies, seem to be developing. If exercises are selected in which group members are asked to choose partners, you learn a lot and can map the choices and the changes as the group develops over the weeks.

When open conflict arises, or members are obviously excited by or particularly interested in certain subjects, this is easy to record, but the teacher is perhaps less apt to record topics that seem to bore them or that do not result in questions and further discussion. Yet data on this is highly relevant.

So the beginning of working with groups is *observing* and *learning* from them, and this has to go hand in hand with counselling, providing information, broaching new topics, and stimulating members of the group to seek more. Before we can teach we must learn from the women themselves. They have a great deal to give us. In learning from them their ideas about their bodies and birth, about family relationships and the things they worry about or hope or fear, we shall have a basis for understanding which will permit us to adapt our teaching to answer their needs.

Helping Underprivileged Mothers in Groups

On the whole it is probably safe to say that mothers from lower socioeconomic groups and those from non-Western cultures are much more concerned to be good mothers than at getting control over their bodies in labour, at being in command of the situation, escaping social humiliation in childbirth or fearing ridicule in exposing aspects of their personality which are crude, vulgar or shameful. Many of the things that educated women worry about concern not only pain or laceration but feelings of helplessness, inferiority and losing face. They are afraid that they may say things to the doctor that they never really intended, revealing their own dark thoughts or a hidden streak of vulgarity. They are often afraid that they will scream and weep and 'make a fool of myself'. When they do cry out or groan, and even when they grunt with bearing down, they frequently make elaborate apologies for their childishness or stupidity. Many middle-class women are most worried about what they see as a relapse into infantile dependence; losing control of the bowels and 'dirtying the bed'.

Peasant women and the urban poor seem to have more straightforward attitudes to birth which rarely involve them in such tortured thinking. If one watches peasant women in childbirth they often appear to accept what is happening to their bodies in a more direct way; they may suffer acute pain, may moan and call out to God or cry for their mothers, but they do not interpret their behaviour as a lapse from a normal well-behaved, well-brought up, polite self. There is no idealized self standing as it were, outside themselves and a little apart from them which they look to as their real selves, and hence no feelings of shame and self-recrimination when they find themselves acting in a way different from this exterior, socially approved pattern. This is one reason, perhaps, why even simple rudimentary teaching for childbirth can be especially rewarding with these pupils.

Basically they often seem happier with their bodies and with the maternal function than many women who have had much more education and who seem to have greater advantages in all things. But because they are different they cannot be taught in the same way as one would set about teaching a class of university graduates. Many methods in antenatal education are modelled almost entirely on working with just this sort of woman, because up to now it has been on the whole the schoolteachers and librarians, the psychologists and nurses, and other professional women, who have chosen to come to classes.

I do not intend here to set a blueprint for teaching different types of women, because it is only those actually working in the field themselves who can work out effective methods, but for you who have been working with more privileged mothers it is important to remember that you will get little response if you put all the emphasis on 'handling contractions', on coping with stress, and on maintaining the dignity of womanhood. The emphasis should rather be on good mothering, whether it is the mothering of the baby still in utero, the child in process of being born, the neonate, or that aspect of good mothering which prompts a couple to space their births and plan the family. All these aspects of mothering are interdependent. But there is even more to it than this.

We tend in our teaching to intellectualize childbirth—to turn all those powerful emotional and physiological sensations into mere verbal symbols and, for those not familiar with the symbols or who do not understand their complexity, whether or not they have received formal education, thereby dilute the meanings and render them neutral and colourless. Sometimes we do this almost in spite of ourselves, as if we could not ourselves come face to face with the intensity of the experience of childbirth; we talk hopefully and deceptive about 'discomfort' when we really mean pain; we say 'hard work' when we mean that a woman feels as if she is using her last ounce of strength and is at the limit of endurance; and we talk about maternal feelings as if they involved only a gentle sweetness and not the whole range of human passions. So we can be dishonest when we least intend to be, and something is lost from our teaching: the sense of reality and genuine feelings with which people have to cope.

Perhaps we think that we can thus control these emotions better; and that by not casting a searchlight on them they will not intrude. Such a process of verbalization and intellectualization serves to evade the main issue: that of an overwhelming total psychosexual experience which for many women may be the biggest thing that has ever happened to them—only equal in its intensity and vividness to the experience of falling in love or of sexual passion.

In teaching mothers who have had little or no academic education we should aim to come back to essentials and clear away some of the verbiage and, with this, some of the mechanical exercises which are unrelated to the reality of the experience of labour. Gymnastic drills are irrelevant unless they are of the kind which bring women to a more sensitive awareness of their bodies, which helps them work with them better and assists harmonious psychophysical functioning. Very few purely mechanical drills are of this kind.

There is little point in telling them all about Pavlov and his dogs; they will only wonder what it has to do with them. Avoid especially introducing any pseudomagic concept of 'blocking' pain, which can so easily be incorporated into a preexisting system of magico-religious belief or superstition. Pavlovian psychology is much over-simplified in the way in which it is included in methods of training in psychoprophylaxis, so much so that notions of raising the pain threshold by techniques of distraction and by disassociation can be used as semimagical devices to ward off evil.

In the course of this chapter I have made suggestions which constitute not tricks to get women to retain facts but a method of teaching based on the conviction that the woman in labour is primarily a person—not a functioning uterus linked to a cerebral cortex, for such a partial and distorted view of human behaviour is bound to fail when we try to make it a basis for education for the emotionally significant act of giving birth.

From a sociological point of view, too, the women we teach are each part of a system of social and family relationships—part of a culture. Everything they do and feel is inseparable from the interlocking and interrelated social roles they enact, from their consciousness of their own identity and the bonds they have with others. We cannot afford to neglect these facts of human existence or the manifold facets of personality which, as we understand them better, must affect the way we teach. In effect, therefore, we modify our teaching to suit different types of women and do not promulgate it as a creed which allows no variations in conduct.

There *are* dangers along this road—the dangers of imprecision and muddle—but the dangers from those who teach purely mechanical methods are much greater.

What, in fact, do we really want? I know what I want to do. I want to help each woman to be able to trust her body, and willingly, gladly, with her eyes shining, to give birth. To do this she needs not only technical know-how—though an adequate activity of response to the signal of uterine contractions is important—not only intellectual information but a psychosexual harmony through which she can joyfully surrender her body to the creative experience. This has significance in the moments of birth, for the couple in their marriage, and for relationships within the family and society.

My aim is to help the prospective parents to prepare themselves so that pregnancy and childbirth can be integrated both within the context of their own intimate psychosexual lives, and the capacities for pleasure and for real feelings inherent in those lives, and within the pattern of human relationships represented by marriage, family and the wider society. In this process the antenatal class has great educative and psychotherapeutic potential.

4

Organizing the Classes

Antenatal classes are customarily held during the last trimester of pregnancy, but it is of great advantage to involve expectant mothers much earlier—if for only one class—and with hospital-based classes even at the time of the first clinic appointment if possible. Certainly if one is going to discuss diet and health during pregnancy it is desirable to do this within the first three months.

Classes which take place in the hospital may be best held at times which precede or follow on clinics, when the mother will have had to make the journey to the hospital anyway. If a creche can take care of other children this will free multiparae for attending classes too. It is a great help to have multiparae in the class who can talk of their own personal experiences, and who have practical knowledge of baby care to contribute.

Many teachers working in hospitals will find that they only get patients turning up, perhaps rather nonchalantly, because they have been 'sent' in the last few weeks. This can be very frustrating, but they should be given a warm welcome. It is much better to have them then than not to have them at all. Even when a woman is admitted in early labour it is not too late for a class, and every opportunity should be taken to do the work under the conditions which limit it in that particular hospital.

Ideally one needs about eight group meetings or classes in each course, but at lower ends of the socioeconomic scale if mothers cannot afford bus fares, have the care of other members of the family at home, are put off by what they interpret as patronization or haughty superiority on the part of even one member of the hospital staff, or if they find pregnancy exhausting and are always tired out, there will be times when they do not come. Then it may be a good idea to have home addresses ready, and to write, phone if possible, or better still, if this proves practical, look them up in person, with an invitation to attend the next class. Sometimes when a woman misses one she may feel guilty and think she will not be welcome at the next class.

Between an hour and two hours is usually ample for classes. These should not be divided into practical and theoretical *or* exercises and lectures, but should be one unified whole. Continuity in the running of classes should be ensured at the outset, since nothing is worse than a continual change of teachers. However, informal discussions are extremely helpful—*not*, I believe, lectures—with labour ward staff and others actively involved in antepartum and postpartum care, and with breastfeeding and postnatal support counsellors if they are available in the area; these people should be present throughout at least one class, rather than come in from outside, do their bit, and then go away again. If they stay on after the class individuals can go up and talk casually with them about any specific problems.

Subjects Covered in the Course

Classes should be progressive, and not merely repetitive. A woman should feel each time that she has learned something, seen a subject in a new light, and acquired a little more confidence. This does not mean that completely different topics have to be tackled at each class the first stage being dealt with in one, the second in another, and so on; very few people accurately remember what they have been told the first time. The course should be arranged so that someone missing a class does not feel that she might as well give up because she has missed essential information. I prefer to think of concentric circles, with labour in the middle, and approach the central subject from different points on the periphery relating this also to the antepartum and postpartum periods, to other aspects of everyday life and to other kinds of stress. We might, for instance, explore the subjects of relaxation, rhythm, or breathing, not only of the first stage, transition and delivery but of the changes in pregnancy (What is the rhythm of the baby's movements in utero like?) or how a mother holds her baby at the breast and the rhythm of its sucking. In this way the same topics are approached in varying contexts.

Classes cover the following subjects:

1. As early as possible in pregnancy there should be an opportunity for discussion of the physical and emotional adjustments to pregnancy: diet, rest, good posture and working habits, possible stress in the marriage, smoking and drugs might all be discussed, with group members actively involved not merely listening to a talk.

2. Anatomy and physiology of the reproductive system and the way women *feel* about their bodies and how they imagine them to be. Pain and our attitudes to it.

3. Fetal development; old wives' tales; fears and apprehensions.

4. The course of normal labour; the prelabour phase, signs of labour, first stage, transition, second and third stages, and the appearance and care of the newborn baby.

5. Drugs, hospital routines, fetal monitoring, sonar scanning, midwifery terms and procedures,* and how to cooperate and communicate with labour attendants.

6. The emotional and physical stresses of labour.

7. Variations on usual patterns of labour (that is, not abnormal labours), including induction, occipito-posterior, breech, placenta praevia, delivery *with the help of* forceps or ventouse, Caesarean section, trials of labour, and any problems faced by members of the class or others about which they have heard.

8. General breathing awareness and control, linked with progressive relaxation, members of the group working together.

9. Differential relaxation of the face, throat, shoulders, chest,

---

* See Margaret Williams and Dorothy Booth, *Antenatal Education: Guidelines for Teachers* (Edinburgh, Churchill Livingstone, 1974) and note their cogent comments on 'VX', 'cephal' and F-NH.

limbs, buttocks, abdomen, and the like and awareness and control of the pelvic floor. The teacher helps pupils to become conscious of the contraction and release of specific muscle groups by using the method of Touch Relaxation, some Stanislavsky-based exercises, and some Jacobson techniques. You move around the room in close contact and active relation with them.

10. Breathing techniques for labour. Simulated contractions, using manual squeezing on the inner thigh, of varying intensity and length, working in pairs or as husband/wife teams. Problems of hyperventilation, and what to do about it.

11. Relaxation and breathing used for adjustment to the successive phases of the first and second stages of labour, and adaptive techniques for the transition phase between the first and second stages.

12. Pushing for maximum efficiency without straining, and breathing for delivery.

13. Comfortable and mechanically useful positions and movements. Massage: abdominal, sacrolumbar, shoulder and upper back, buttocks, inner thigh and leg. Backache in labour. Fatigue in the long labour. Problems of the precipitate labour and of pharmacologically induced and accelerated labours.

14. How the husband can help both in pregnancy and the puerperium and during the first and second stages of labour.

15. Labour rehearsal to build up a pattern of response to the stimuli of uterine contractions, using manual squeezing.

16. Postnatal emotional and physical adjustment. The maintenance of correct postural tone in the puerperium, rehabilitation of the pelvic floor and abdominal muscles. Reduction of puerperal stress, both physical and emotional.

17. The relationship of both parents with the new baby and each other. Feeding and *parenting* (Yes, it used to be called mothercraft, but this is rather more to the point). The problems of fatigue, depression and anxiety. Relatives, neighbours, friends, professional advisers, the advice and help they give. The displaced sibling and jealousy. Postnatal sexual adjustment, and birth control.

This material can be spread over six to ten classes with, if possible, a private consultation too, however short it must be.

The Room and Its Equipment

The physical environment of the class affects its atmosphere and its potential in obvious ways. Classes should be held in a clean, warm but airy, well-ventilated and, above all, quiet room, not overlooked by other buildings (or with adequate curtaining or blinds if this is inevitable), with soft, indirect lighting and, if possible, pleasant colours and furnishings. Lying on the floor and staring up into centrally placed light bulbs is not conducive to relaxation. For this reason a large sitting room is often much better than a clinic room or one kept specially for that purpose. (In my own home I sometimes use a very big bedroom, which has a lofty beamed ceiling and brilliant hangings round the fourposter bed and at the windows. I wondered whether pupils would mind being asked to meet in the bedroom, but have discovered that they enjoy it because it is comfortable and colourful. In summer we might meet out in the garden, and cushions and rugs are spread on the lawn near the roses.)

Whether teaching in a public building or in one's own home, magazines, books, paintings, flowers and a few comfortable chairs so that women can learn how to relax sitting, not only lying on the floor, all add to the picture of relaxed friendliness. On the floor there should be a thick carpet or rugs. Each woman should have ample room to stretch herself lying full length, and to turn over and adjust her position (although I realize that this is often a counsel of perfection). Interruptions must be kept to the minimum, and it may be a good idea to switch off the telephone. The lavatory should be easily available and should be fresh and clean (and this can be quite difficult to ensure when there are young children in the house). All soft furnishings, pillows and pillowslips should be clean.

In hospitals, classes should be held on fairly neutral territory. A big, bare gymnasium is quite unsuitable and is often accoustically impossible. Consider where women will wait, for the atmosphere in which they do so may be an important factor in their willing acceptance or rejection of classes. Nothing can be more depressing than sitting on rows of hard benches with blank doors and a pile of dirty, dog-eared and out-of-date magazines, while obviously very sick patients drag themselves through the corridors. Even in the waiting area, if chairs can be grouped so that women can talk together and find out about each other, the informal, spontaneously created subgroups thus established may form a valuable adjunct to the class.

If possible have visual aids available in the waiting area, not only posters and pictures but, for example, a videotape machine which, at the press of a button, shows fetal development, health during pregnancy, new baby care, or birth. But, as we shall see when discussing audio-visual equipment, such aids should always be shown within a context of teaching, and it is not enough to show material without integrating it within a progressive system of teaching. Unless integrated in this way visual aids can shock, titillate, confuse, or entertain, without educating.

However, it would be a pity if anyone were put off teaching because they did not possess these ideal conditions. Anywhere is better than nowhere, and any waiting room or open space suitably screened in hospital or health centre can, with some imagination, be utilized. If it is difficult to make a quiet corner in the hospital, or the room available is much too large, rolls of corrugated cardboard approximately 183 cm (6 ft) wide can be used to portion off a space for the class, and can easily be stored in a cupboard when not in use.

Focal points in the room should be kept fairly low, and one can distract even from lofty ceilings or windows set high in the wall by switching off ceiling lights and having pools of light from ordinary table lamps set around the space available for the group. A few inexpensive lamps and a bunch of flowers can make even the starkest room look welcoming.

Sometimes there is insufficient space for all women to lie down and practise relaxation and comfortable positions for labour. Then half the class may be able to lie on the mats while the others assist them, test their relaxation and help with their breathing. There is a positive advantage in this arrangement, since they can move about, be actively involved, feel each other's limbs, so that they know exactly what happens when a muscle contracts, learn how to correct each other's mistakes, share problems and have a sense of comrade-ship. If only a handful of women can lie down at any one time, one can still have a class. It should be noted in passing that the teacher should aim to have sufficient space, and a fan, open windows or air conditioning for good ventilation, as many women perspire heavily in late pregnancy and many also become acutely sensitive to odours, which can trigger off nausea. (For the same reason, you should be careful of your own personal hygiene, so that, however busy you are you are always clean, fresh-smelling and well-groomed.)

Few teachers will have all they desire in the way of classrooms. But they can determine to be adaptable and to use the limiting conditions as opportunities for experiment.

Ideally one teacher works with not more than sixteen women, or seven to eight couples, allowing face-to-face communication and direct person-to-person continuing relationships over a series of classes. Group members should be able not only to hear each other but to see each other's faces without having to turn or tense up. They all get to know each other and have an opportunity, perhaps, to talk together before or after the class.

Teaching in one's own home provides the best situation for friendly hospitality and relationships of this kind. In many hospitals and clinics one is reduced to having women drop in either out of curiosity or because they have to wait around to see the doctor, or to having audiences, rather than classes, of thirty women or so. If the only way to teach in a particular hospital is to do it this way, grasp the opportunity and take thirty women. Project your voice and your personality and develop techniques which suit the situation. These are bound to be different from techniques which grow out of working with small groups. Working under difficult conditions like this your first task is to be audible, and you will have to use large gestures and dramatize your material in no uncertain terms. But it can be done!

Pillows

One foam wedge (61 cm [2 ft] square, sloping from 20 cm [8 in] to 7 cm [3 in] is a good size) and three or four firm foam or terylene pillows covered attractively, and kept freshly laundered, should be available for each woman, with the addition of a plastic covered bolster stuffed with foam chips or in Britain a Hexham inflatable polythene bolster* under the knees in the dorsal position to help easy relaxation of the abdominal muscles. The Hexham bags can also be used, not too firmly inflated, behind women's backs and under the upper leg and beneath the head in the front lateral position, where storage facilities for equipment are inadequate.

Pupils should also be able to relax, however, without cushions under the knees, since some hospitals object to their use in labour, believing that they will reduce circulation of the blood in the legs of an immobile patient. The woman in labour should not be immobile, but encouraged to change position frequently and to talk about if she feels like it. (When a woman is relatively immobilized by a drip it is good for her to move her legs now and again. I suggest that she exercises her feet in between contractions, and draws the letters of the alphabet with each foot alternately. The variety of letter shapes makes the task more likely to be performed than if she is told just to 'wiggle her toes'.)

Small cushions and foam off-cuts are helpful for the small of the back in the dorsal position and for under the breasts and the upper leg in the lateral position. In the dorsal position, which is useful in class, as teacher and students can see each other's faces more easily, the wedge, bolsters and pillows are used to ensure good support right up the back, including the head, neck and shoulders. Remember that *no* part of the back should be left unsupported, and the back should be gently rounded, not hollowed. All limbs are well flexed. It is not enough to place support under a pupil's knees. The teacher must ensure that they are resting right on it, with the legs flopped apart and relaxed, and the knees rolled outwards. In fact, your first task in every class is to move around helping pupils to get comfortable, and this personal attention is an important aspect of your relation with them.

* These are designed on the same lines as buoyancy bags in sailing dinghies and, since they can be kept flat when not blown up, are useful when there is little room to store cushions for class use. Details can be obtained from the National Childbirth Trust, 9 Queensborough Terrace, London, W2.

An alternative to a number of pillows and foam supports is to have one solid chair-shaped structure with a couple of pillows as optional extras. The Kitzinger-Sylvester back support was designed for me by an architect/furniture designer, working with a thirty-eight-week pregnant woman, and moulding foam to the curve of her back. This is a useful way of providing firm cushioning in both pregnancy and labour. It is similar to a moulded foam easy chair back, is without a seat or arms, and is covered in stretch towelling which can be easily changed. It can be used both for the first stage and for delivery, providing back support for the woman in a well-rounded, upright, semisquatting position.

To relate practice positions to labour, when the woman is able to use these during labour or have similar sorts of support, we should explain that during the earlier part of the first stage many women are happy moving around, but once they are more comfortable on a bed, the wedge (with the 5 cm (2 in) edge under the buttocks) and bolster can be used. From the late first stage, or from when contractions are lasting about one minute and are coming every two to four minutes, if a wedge is allowed it may be most comfortable to reverse it, so that the 20 cm (8 in) edge is under the buttocks. With this support a woman can adopt a semisquatting or sitting position in labour with equal comfort. In domiciliary deliveries this wedge can be used for delivery.

Once the baby's head is on the perineum and can be seen during contractions the bolster is removed. The buttocks should be exactly on the 20 cm (8 in) edge of the wedge. The shoulders are rounded forward, the chin on the chest during bearing down. The mother is able to watch the crowning of the baby's head and the subsequent birth if she wishes, and seeing it helps her to control her actions during these important moments. The advantage to the midwife is that the baby does not descend into a pool of liquor or a dip in the mattress. It also facilitates delivery of the anterior shoulder should the baby be large.

If the woman who is to be delivered in hospital will not have these pillows in labour, it is pointless rehearsing her exclusively under more comfortable conditions, and she should practise frequently with the equipment with which she will be provided.

Teaching Aids

Obviously personality differences in teaching techniques involve preferences in audio-visual aids, and every teacher may use the material a little differently. The aim in each case is to make the actual rehearsal for labour more vivid and real to the expectant mother, so that she does not finally find herself confronted with a physiological and emotional experience for which she is completely unprepared. If we keep this aim in mind we shall find that certain sorts of material, which might be useful with medical students or pupil midwives, will be of no help to the mothers in our care. Their very lack of aesthetic appeal may make it more difficult for the mother to adjust to her labour without reservations, and cause the kind of 'holding back', so quickly translated into muscular tension, which tends to make labour longer and more difficult.

Films are the most dramatic way of introducing the expectant mother and father to the facts of birth. But too often these sophisticated aids are used in a teaching vacuum, without adequate introduction or preparation of the intended audience. I remember one large American hospital where video-tapes were shown in the waiting-room of the antenatal clinic, and any woman entering only had to press a button to see a full and splendid, vividly coloured Caesarean section.

Sometimes, too, films are shown without the people introducing them having ever seen them themselves, so that they can be non-plussed when it comes to questions or to leading a discussion following the showing. Because something is made into a film this does not mean that it is the best way of demonstrating it; nor because it is made into a film does it follow that it is correct or that the facts illustrated will be interpreted accurately by the audience. A case in point is depicting a ripe ovum as a large circular object about the size of a tennis ball. I have known women reject this information out of hand because, as they correctly asserted, they did not have anything that size coming out halfway between two periods, so they were sure it did not happen to them. One sex education film, parts of which are intended to be diagrammatic, while other frames are realistic, shows an enormous penis in bright green.

Some films, which attempt to put over moral ideas as well as facts, link birth with the beauties of nature and the tenderness of love and can prove hilarious to an audience which is not in the right mood for this or is not accustomed to thinking in such terms. Others can shock and bombard with facts for which the audience is not ready. Particularly is this so of colour films of birth in which episiotomy or the delivery of the placenta is lovingly lingered over or in which there is a good deal of bleeding. Blood is never so red as in a colour film of delivery!

American films in which the labouring woman is shown heavily swathed in sterile drapes, legs in lithotomy and wrists handcuffed, surrounded by inexplicable machines, gleaming steel and officiating medical and nursing staff dressed up to look like something out of the Ku Klux Klan, can be terrifying for people coming from rural backgrounds in which birth is a family event and one that normally takes place at home, or even for women who are not accustomed to all the trappings of a large teaching hospital. On the other hand, when I showed a fairly sophisticated American audience an English birth film, I realized that in actually putting on view a woman's whole perineum and vulva I was submitting them to a possibly shocking experience, because in American obstetrics the female body in parturition is completely depersonalized. An English birth film then becomes something of a blue movie. If in American films designed to show happy deliveries, the mother is shown displaying delight at the birth, the expression on her face takes place at the other end of the great divide between the birth-giving vulva, which has been appropriated by the obstetrician, and the person who feels emotion.

It is within this culture context that American doctors may find it hard to see that, whereas for their patients it can be disturbing to see a baby actually emerging from a vagina, to many others it looks equally peculiar and distasteful to see a baby being born through a hole in a white or green sheet and not, apparently, out of a woman's body at all. The kind of film which is most useful is *Birth*; a film about feelings and experiences in which different types of women describe their varying experiences of labour and two deliveries are shown in the context of the relationship between the couple and the welcome the new parents give to the baby.*

Films must be used with care and should never be shown before adequate preparation has paved the way for understanding of what they are all about. Film strips and slides can be useful in that the teacher can adapt whatever she is talking about to suit that particular audience. Moreover some slides may be quickly dealt with or omitted altogether, and more time spent on others.

There is a disadvantage in not having the group meeting room well-lit and being able to see into their faces, and they into yours. Once a group is seated in front of a screen it becomes an audience rather than a participating group, and in those classes which can meet only a few times, or in which the membership is always changing—both of which can happen in large clinic departments—this may be too great a price to pay. With all other aids, except when there is a very large number in the class, it can usually be arranged that women sit in a half or full circle. They can move if necessary to see more clearly any particular teaching aids, and the very moving around can add to the informality and friendliness of the occasion. The teacher can use difficulties of space or lighting to draw the group closer together and to get the women further involved. You can ask a woman to hold up a poster for the others to see or to pass round some photographs, and in this way help women to feel that they are not only recipients of information but participants in the teaching process and sharing responsibility. The shyer and more uncommunicative the group, the more important these techniques are. For this reason, if for no other, teaching aids which do not involve darkening a room or seating women in rows may be the most appropriate.

Photographs and drawings of posture in pregnancy, of labour and about postnatal rehabilitation, and those in *The Birth Atlas, A Baby is Born*† and *The First Nine Months of Life*,‡ can be extremely useful

*National Childbirth Trust, 9 Queensborough Terrace, London W2.

† Both published by the New York Maternity Center, 48 East 92nd Street, New York, N.Y. 10028. The latter is published in Britain by Allen & Unwin, 1966.

‡ Geraldine Lux Flanagan (London, Heinemann, 1963).

and compelling material. If these can be supplemented by large photographs of mothers in labour, and particularly during delivery, they can do much to reeducate the woman away from the association of labour with inevitable ugliness, suffering and horror. As we make plans for more photographs of this type it must be remembered that a string of pearls, earrings, a pretty nightdress, a hair ribbon on the mother, or flowers in the background can all help in this process.

Photographs, including those of babies born to previous members of the class, birth photographs and others should include as many as possible which are obviously of people like those in the group, with racial and other characteristics with which they can identify. Avoid with care the sort of illustration copiously available in booklets put out by baby-food manufacturers in which a golden-haired mother— obviously a model—dressed in a frilly negligée, leans over a lace-trimmed cot; for even a golden-haired mother herself may not identify with this image after a night during which the baby has woken three times for a feed, or in which she is rushing to get a husband off to work with three other children under her feet. This may be what she *should* be like, but she is not. It is very easy for new mothers to feel guilty and to feel they are not measuring up to the standards set not only by their own mothers and older women but by all the advertisements and magazine articles they see: prenatal classes can prepare them for these feelings rather than adding to them.

Charts and diagrams have their uses and their inherent dangers. They are especially liked by expectant fathers, but they tend to systematize that which cannot be subjected to dogmatic simplification. They leave out of account all the modifications and subtle adjustments of technique learned during pregnancy which form part of the pattern of nearly every labour. A woman in labour does not work like a motor-car engine, however much some enthusiasts among antenatal teachers have tried to draw analogies of this kind.

In fixing our eyes on oversimplified charts and diagrams we are in danger of losing sight of the woman as an individual. Sometimes it has even been suggested that a woman should have charts of respiration near her on the wall to consult actually during her labour. We should rather aim at her being able to relate herself to the inner activity coming from her contracting uterus. To seek any other focus of attention is merely to distract and evade the psychophysical adjustment which is the basis of all harmonious activity, whether it be riding a bicycle, swimming, playing the piano, making love, or having a baby.

Teaching aids involving three-dimensional materials should be explored more fully. In some societies people are unaccustomed to see flat pictures. They are used to handling things in the round, to dealing with tangible objects, but not to looking at books or films, or sometimes even magazines or drawings. This is particularly true of peasant societies. It is also true of those societies in which formal education is minimal, and where only a minority read and write with any comprehension. The totally unfamiliar can be an assault on the senses, so that the meaning which it is intended to convey is lost. Even with women who are familiar with the written word and with pictorial illustrations the occasional use of ordinary objects which they are used to handling can provide a much better visual aid than more complicated aids specially designed for the purpose. Ordinary kitchen tools and equipment and the ingredients of fridge and larder can come in useful. Even if you do not want actually to illustrate the process of bearing down in the second stage of labour by using a pastry bag and stiff egg white, the verbal illustration in itself can be apposite. In peasant societies with women accustomed to working on the land or selling the produce, the familiar shapes of fruit and vegetables can form a useful comparison with the anatomical forms which you want to illustrate.

An avocado pear provides an excellent illustration of the uterus in early pregnancy. Turning the stalk end downwards the teacher can explain that this is how it lies in a woman's body, that this part is called the cervix, and it hangs down into the vagina, like the clapper of a bell. The uterus has only one opening, downwards, and the baby cannot come out of the belly, abdomen (or whatever term is normally used by the women you are teaching); it can only come down. The size of the uterus at term can be demonstrated with a marrow, or squash, again with the stalk end down, and the teacher can explain how the walls have thinned out, that of course really the uterus is a hollow muscle, not solid like an avocado or marrow, and show, perhaps with the aid of a tied water-filled polythene bag of corresponding size, the bag of waters, and with an easily flexed doll, the way in which the baby nestles inside, curled up into a ball. When discussing moulding of the fetal head a soft grapefruit can be similarly useful.

The New York Maternity Center's pattern for a knitted uterus is also useful, with layers of elasticated thread sewn through the cervix, a balloon blown up inside the uterus, and a ball between the balloon and the cervix. Pressing gently on the balloon (*do not* let the uterus rupture!) forces the ball into the cervix, and gradually thins it out and dilates it. For some women the knitted uterus is incomprehensible, however, and to others it seems merely ludicrous; so it should be used with discretion, and always only after prior practice.

Beware, however, the overprecise use of comparisons of function when these can give rise to inaccuracies. In discussing the process of osmosis which takes place in the placenta, the image of a coffee percolator is indeed useful, if one does not extend the comparison too far. We certainly do not want to leave even one woman with the impression that the contents of her uterus are at a bubbling boil, that the liquor is coffee-colour, or that she must consume large quantities of coffee to make this process work. So it may help to use more than one relevant image and to refer also to 'a plant with its roots in the soil, rather as the placenta sends out roots into the lining of the uterus' and to the structure of the placenta 'like a sponge with little holes through which the blood can flow'. Be careful to add that it does not look like the clean pink sponge you have in your hand, but more like a large piece of raw liver.

Women in the classes may themselves introduce new images which can be useful, and you should always be ready to incorporate these into your teaching and to have an ear tuned to them.

Some exercises are helpful teaching aids for instruction in anatomy and physiology. Perhaps the most useful is a bare, flat wall against which exercises for posture can be done; the firmness of the wall can lead to an appreciation of the movement of the spine, and increased ability to stand with a straight back. Cheap kitchen candles can be lit and used for breathing exercises which can be useful for women who breathe shallowly or who lack breathing control. The game is to blow on the flame without putting it out, and yet keep it flickering.

The most vivid teaching aid, and the most adaptable, is probably a soft, cuddly doll of correct new-baby proportions. Any doll used for antenatal teaching should conform to four criteria:

It should be attractive to look at, so that mothers can easily identify their babies with the one in the teacher's arms. Ordinary demonstration fetuses for pupil midwives are nightmare monstrosities liable to nourish any fantasies the expectant mother may have about bearing a deformed baby.

It should be as nearly as possible like a real newborn baby in appearance and size.

It must be flexible (this entails a cloth body).

And it ought to be pleasant to handle.

After a long search some years ago I found a suitable doll and devised what has come to be known as the *box pelvis*, or *baby box*, to go with it, and some techniques of demonstration. The box is an ordinary circular plastic kitchen container, with an oval cut out to indicate the dimensions of the pelvic outlet, and two layers of foam with a slit down the centre are glued over the opening to represent the perineum. The slit is rounded off in the centre to represent the vagina.

To the doll I attach three strands of plastic-covered electric flex twisted round each other and sewn into the abdomen to represent the umbilical cord, and to the end of this I attach a foam rubber sponge to represent the placenta.

Teachers should always handle the doll gently and carefully, for to the mothers in the class this is their baby. It should never be thrown down, twisted roughly or even discarded abruptly. It is best for it to have a basket of its own, where it can be kept with other teaching aids, such as the knitted uterus and a sock and ball to indicate the curve of the birth canal through which the baby's head passes.

Demonstration 1

Using your own body and standing up indicate lie and attitude. Talk about the different positions in which the baby may be lying during pregnancy, encouraging pupils to discuss this, their feelings about it, the baby's movements, and if necessary, their fears. Demonstrate flexion and extension of the fetal spine, head and limbs. All the time you have the doll in your hands and clearly demonstrate the different positions.

Demonstration 2

Using your own body, discuss *presentation*.* Illustrate vertex and breech presentations. Discuss flexion and extension of breeches. This can be demonstrated in terms of flexed breech, but not quite so clearly for an extended breech as the doll's legs are probably fixed in partial flexion and do not adequately splint the spine; but this can be explained. Discuss and illustrate anterior and posterior presentations of the vertex, encouraging mothers near term to feel their own abdomens; discuss where the baby kicks, and relate this to indications of presentation such as a saucer-shaped depression round the mother's umbilicus and dispersed kicking movements all over the abdomen typical of posteriors. When the mothers are shown the doll as an occipito-posterior and as an anterior they can relate themselves in a more satisfying way to the actual movements and position of their own babies.

The teacher should, however, always emphasize the normal, however interested the class becomes in deviations from the normal.

Demonstration 3

Demonstrate the size and shape of the pelvic outlet. Discuss the concertina-like flexibility of the tissues of the birth canal, the action of hormones in the bloodstream in pregnancy on tissues and ligaments, and show sponge perineum and vagina. (Allow opportunity for amusement at this, and share in it.)

Follow this by demonstrating usual sequence of events during

　* See *Experience of Childbirth* (Pelican ed.).

second stage.* You now have to act two parts, that of the mother bearing the child and that of the midwife or obstetrician, and differentiate clearly between the actions of the two as you proceed.

Sit, with the baby flexed on your lap, the occiput presenting, and demonstrate breathing for expulsion, whilst yourself bearing down, your hand inside the box supporting the head and allowing it gradually to dilate the vagina. As the head crowns you stop pushing and 'breathe the baby out'. Both strong and gentle pushing should be demonstrated, and the likely effects of 'blowing away' a contraction when necessary. Discuss what might happen if the head pops out 'like a cork out of a champagne bottle'.

Demonstrate both left occipito-anterior and right occipito-anterior and subsequent external rotation of the head.

Discuss episiotomy and show where and when it may be performed. If the group is interested follow this with discussion of aids to comfortable intercourse when there is soreness in the postnatal period.

Guarding of the perineum can be demonstrated and other techniques of delivery, not only from the mother's point of view but in terms of how she may help the midwife or obstetrician control and assist delivery. Demonstrate delivery of wide shoulders, what is done when the cord is around the neck, suction and cutting of the cord.

Demonstration 4

Introduce discussion about posterior and breech presentations by saying that you will show them some of the less usual positions in which the baby may lie. Discuss occipito-posterior presentations and the usual progress of labour when the head rotates. Then demonstrate persistent occipito-posterior delivery (make sure the perineum will allow delivery of the doll in this way, since it is much more of a strain on the foam, and it would be unfortunate if, in demonstrating, the teacher ripped the 'mother' to pieces!). If confident in your obstetric skill you may even demonstrate the delivery of a face

* Visually the effect is similar to that of my drawings on page 34 of *The Experience of Childbirth* (Pelican ed.).

presentation and discuss the effect on the baby's face; consider also demonstrating the difficulty of a brow presentation and show what is done about it.

Demonstrate the kind of breech delivery commonly used in hospitals in the area. Act the mother's part, showing what she may be required to do, and discuss what she feels before and during the birth of the body for example, and a nonexistent or very confused urge to push. Discuss why speedy but carefully controlled delivery of the after-coming head is important. Always conclude each demonstration of delivery of a breech with resuscitation of the baby, so that the mother expects and is not shocked by it.

Demonstration 5

Discuss placenta praevia and demonstrate partial and complete placenta praevia. Discuss APH and Caesarean section in this context.

Demonstration 6

In order not to overemphasize manipulations involved in delivery and thus encourage the mother to lose trust in her own body, demonstrate what to do if one is all alone and having a baby. Demonstrate spontaneous delivery with minimum push technique bearing down (that is, mouth-centred light rapid breathing with the breath held only when the urge to do so is compelling). Show natural expulsion of baby without handling, tilted position of newborn baby to facilitate drainage of mucus, and how the cord is usually long enough for the baby to be put to the breast immediately so that placental separation is encouraged.

Demonstrations can, of course, be in any order according to the classes' requirements and their questions. Some will merge with or follow immediately on others. But always stress the normal and leave the class with the normal in their minds, however fascinating the mechanics of the abnormal.

Let the mothers handle the doll themselves and practise delivery if they wish. They will begin also to appreciate some of the skills of the good obstetrician or midwife, and this is important for their cooperation in labour. To this end it is important not to construct the perineum too slackly, as birth is then so easy that manipulation becomes irrelevant. The delivery of the head by a process of extension as it slides over the perineum should follow mechanically as the easiest process during delivery of the doll, and this does in fact occur, it being almost impossible to get the head through the opening in any other way.

The demonstration model is particularly useful with husbands, and especially with the rather apprehensive ones. Most men greatly appreciate the mechanics of delivery and like to be instructed about them. In cases where a breech delivery with the husband present is anticipated, careful instruction can prepare him completely.

Records and tape recordings are most useful when preparation is already well under way, not because they overstimulate but because to women accustomed to the refinements of audio-visual stimulus from television, they are inadequate unless the woman already has a context with which to relate the information she is acquiring. The tape recording of a labour can be very useful in a class as an integral part of the preparation for labour if the women use the adaptive respiratory and other techniques at the same time, and act their way through the labour. They must remember, for instance, to 'breathe the baby out' at the appropriate time, and need adequate coaching from the teacher as labour progresses. Such 'acting through' a labour (described more fully on page 8) can be a therapeutic experience and one which relates them to the actuality of labour in an intense and effective way. Tapes more than any other teaching aids are culture-bound, at the same time demanding an effort of concentration on the part of the women too great for those who may feel that these are just not their sort of people, nor the sort of things they would be saying when having a baby. I would, therefore, not include tape recordings as useful teaching aids when working with other cultural groups.

The sounds which may be heard by the baby in utero and which are recorded on Dr Hajime Murooka cassette tape called *Lullaby from the Womb* (also available as a record) are a very effective way of initiating discussion about the baby's intrauterine environment and as a basis for talking about the baby not just as an 'it' but as a person. Couples practising together at home also value the opportunity to use a tape recording which means that they can concentrate on relaxation, breathing and massage, for instance, without having continually to turn the pages of a book. Such a cassette tape can also be very useful for couples who cannot get to classes, as well as for student teachers wishing to 'tune in' to a more experienced teacher's style and the way in which she expresses herself in teaching. For these reasons, my own two hours' recording, *Journey through Birth*,* may be helpful.

There is one thing which you as the teacher can be using all of the time, however, and it is by far the most valuable teaching aid: your *own body*. You use it every time you speak, not only with gesture and facial expression but with the very movement of your eyes and the way in which you draw in the group participants. When you talk about breathing, illustrate it with your *own* breathing. When you discuss posture and body mechanics, immediately demonstrate what you are talking about. When you explain relaxation and neuromuscular control, show how your own arm goes 'soft and floppy', or how your neck and shoulder muscles are tight. When you tell about pushing the baby out you too bear down and let the members of the group feel, with a hand against the lower abdomen, how you press the abdominal wall down and forward.

In all this you need to be spontaneous and unselfconscious; if you reflect about what you are doing to the extent of becoming embarrassed the movements become rigid and mechanical. You can be fat or thin, beautiful or ugly—none of this matters—but you must be spontaneous. You should determine never to stand behind a lectern or to sit statistically on a chair; you need to move, to express what you are feeling and describing as vividly as you possibly can. If you can dispense with uniform this is valuable, because not only can it create a barrier of social distance between teacher and pupils, but you need to wear clothes which move easily with your movements.

If you can do all this in a lively way you will find that you can

* Julian Aston Publications, 24 Ladbroke Gardens, London, W11; the National Childbirth Trust; and in the United States: ICEA, 14423 S.E. 23rd Pl. Bellevue, Washington, D.C. 98007.

also use the group's laughter both for the release of tension and as a shared pleasurable experience which can itself be important in the building up of a group feeling of identity. You may be showing an exercise, and add 'not like this', and they laugh, because they can all do it better than *that!*

Teachers who feel that this is their great stumbling point—and this is not surprising, since such skills are rarely taught as part of either teacher or nurse training—might with advantage go to drama lessons. It may be an unanticipated expense in the childbirth education programme, but one that would pay off!

One's body can also be used to illustrate anatomical and physiological material, with the very movement of extended arms and fingers illustrating the action by which the ovum travels along the fallopian tubes into the main body of the uterus (in this case, one's trunk); or the shortening and thickening of the longitudinal muscle fibres of the uterus as the cervix is progressively shortened and dilated; or the movement of the baby's head like a fist moving down the curve of the opposite arm, or under a pubic arch formed from the spread thumb and first finger of the other hand. The possibilities are numerous. If one just stops and imagines that some members of the class are hard of hearing and asks oneself how the material can be demonstrated without relying on words, such mimetic actions will evolve quite easily. I found myself developing a repertoire of this kind in response to a situation in which I actually had a deaf woman in class, to be followed, shortly after, by a Spanish woman who spoke no English, and I am grateful to these pupils for having provided the challenge the response to which was new teaching techniques.

Among the best audio-visual aids concerning new baby care are mothers and babies. Women can be encouraged to come back to the group with their babies, and discussion and demonstration of holding, feeding, changing and bathing babies can proceed with them actually there. The teacher must also here abrogate the role of the expert and let the mothers tell how *they* manage and what *they* find works. We need to be sensitive to the adjustments which these women have to make to the requirements of the family, and if we are teaching underprivileged women, to the particular cultural setting and to the often restricted space and impoverished conditions in their homes. It is no good telling a mother to wash her nipples before feeding the baby if the only water supply is out on a landing, if it is contaminated, or if she then wipes her nipples on a dirty piece of rag. Much better omit such advice.

Audio-visual aids are *not* crutches. They should never be used as props for weak teaching, but rather as means of giving full expression to teaching which is already effective. If you are only just starting out on the road to gaining self-confidence and the individual approach which expresses your skills and personality, it is preferable to concentrate on using your own voice and body *well* and speaking through them, rather than collecting teaching aids. When you do select, invent or modify such aids for your use, those that are flexible and adaptable to your evolving method are the best to choose. A good teaching aid cannot be measured by price. Instead of permitting you to do things that you could not otherwise do with and through yourself, it should, like the potter's wheel or the artist's brush, provide the means of expressing concepts which are a result of your creative search to teach vividly and in your own particular style.

5

The Use of Language

In antenatal teaching language is one of the most important tools used, and to communicate effectively the teacher needs to enjoy using words. Yet the specialist words of midwifery, physiotherapy, sociology or psychology, all of which provide background information for the teacher, are inappropriate to antenatal teaching, and we have to be able to take the ordinary language we use everyday and make of it something both precise and stimulating. Many of the words we shall select are impressionist, suggesting physical states and mental attitudes. They affect the woman's sense of her own body in the process of childbearing. Sometimes this is the most difficult thing to do. It is deceptively easy to create a smoke screen of words. On the one hand is all the information which the teacher (especially the novice teacher) is eager to impart. On the other, there are expectant mothers, longing to know what labour really feels like, what it is like to bear down, and the sensations they may have as the baby is put to the breast. Words often seem inadequate for describing birth, just as they are inadequate for describing the experience of being in love:

> I wanted to say
> I love you
> In fourteen foreign languages
> But most of all (most
> Difficult of all) in English.*

* Peter Roche, 'Somewhere on the way', *The New Love Poetry* (London, Corgi, 1973).

Antenatal teachers must beware of falling back on the 'foreign languages' of textbooks because they cannot take the trouble, or have not the confidence, to find out how to express what they need to say in the language of everyday. It is in this language that we shall find that we gradually evolve our own teaching vocabulary, for language is nothing if it is not alive.

Imagery

The expectant mother benefits from having a basic vocabulary of technical terms about childbirth. With each group we as teachers shall have to feel our way to see how many such terms are useful. The patient who can ask How far am I dilated? is at a distinct advantage in her relations with doctors and nurses over the one who simply asks Is everything all right?—a request which invites merely a soothing answer lacking in information.

However, avoid simply transposing chunks of information from textbooks, or terminology more suitable for the student midwife or obstetrician, with inadequate explanation or illustration or in such a way that it focuses on the pathological rather than the healthy state. The French obstetricians practising psychoprophylaxis sometimes talk about *verbal asepsis*, which they say is just as important as physical asepsis. It is, perhaps, a negative concept—keeping bacteria and anxiety-producing stimuli at bay rather than using language creatively. But often an instructor who is not accustomed to running antenatal classes will give a lecture to pregnant women and inadvertently use phrases which shock and alarm. One doctor opened a talk with: 'If you make a sagittal section of the corpse of a woman who died in childbirth you will see . . .!'* The subject of rehabilitation of the pelvic floor musculature after childbirth is introduced in another work with 'Your vagina, which will have been greatly stretched during the birth, will never again return to its prebirth dimension' and pregnant women are warned to avoid any baths in the last months 'as this may damage the vagina'. More than one teacher uses the phraseology of equipping oneself with

* I. Velvovsky, K. Platonov, V. Ploticher and E. Shugom, *Painless Childbirth through Psychoprophylaxis* (Moscow, Foreign Languages Publishing House, 1960).

techniques as *weapons* for labour, and the birth as *B-Day*, thereby implying that childbirth is a battle which has to be won, rather than a natural process. I always remember my own doctor examining me in late pregnancy, finding twins, and remarking 'I think I can feel two heads' rather than suggesting that she thought there were two *babies* there. A physiotherapist friend who is an antenatal teacher recalls with horror that she used to talk about the fetal head 'hitting' the perineum in the second stage.

Use words which avoid negative suggestion, and select those which reinforce a positive image of the healthy human body in childbirth. This does not mean talking down to mothers. It means that we should illustrate what we are saying as vividly as possible by analogy, simile and metaphor (provided it is understood that it *is* a metaphor) and with the visual aids which we feel we can handle best.

In teaching about the anatomy and physiology of the female reproductive organs, for instance, if you talk about the uterus as it is described in an obstetric textbook, it would be completely inappropriate for prospective parents. Suppose the lesson is about the uterus at term. The teacher who depends too much on a textbook might say:

In late pregnancy the uterus is a large muscular sac with thin, soft, easily compressible walls. This makes the corpus indentable, and enables the fetus to be palpated by the examining fingers. The walls of the uterus are so malleable that the uterus changes shape easily and markedly to accommodate itself to changes in fetal size and position. . . . During pregnancy the cervix becomes progressively softer. This is caused by increased vascularity, general edema, and hyperplasia of the glands. The compound tubular glands become overactive and produce large quantities of mucus. In the cervical canal the secretion accumulates and thickens to form the so-called mucous plug. This inspissated mucus effectively seals off the canal from the vagina, and prevents the ascent of bacteria and other substances into the uterine cavity. . . . At the end of gestation and during labor the internal os gradually disappears, and the cervical canal also becomes part of the lower uterine segment, leaving only the external os.[*]

[*] Harry Oxorn and William R. Foote, *Human Labor & Birth*, 2nd ed. (London, Butterworths, New York, Appleton-Century-Crofts, 1968). This is a useful reference book for the antenatal teacher.

which probably sounds to the expectant mother as if the lesson is about a rather peculiar system of sewage disposal (using the inland waterways perhaps), instead of being intimately concerned with the workings of her body.

The teacher might choose to say something like: 'Although it started off about the size of a fig, by the end of pregnancy the uterus is the size and shape of a harvest festival marrow.' Moreover, the teacher will not simply be saying the words, but will be indicating the pre-pregnancy size with a clenched fist when mentioning the fig, and then will make the shape of the uterus at term with both hands as if slowly feeling its dimensions.

The uterus is an enormous hollow bag of muscle with the baby inside in its bag of waters. The baby is floating inside there in its own private sea, kept at a comfortably warm temperature and cushioned from bumps and bangs by the liquid too. By this time the walls of the uterus have stretched and become thinner and they are about half an inch thick. In the cervix, rather like the cork in the neck of a bottle, is a plug of mucus which seals the contents from the outside world, and from any possible infection. Changes take place in your cervix near the time when the baby is due. It gets really soft, there's more blood flowing to it, it gets a bit puffy, and even before labour starts for many women it starts being drawn up into the uterus a bit, so that, in effect, the neck of the bottle gets shorter. You can probably see this without too much trouble if you squat over a well-lit magnifying mirror—perhaps your husband's got a shaving mirror or you have a make-up mirror like this—and part the labia and look inside. You see, the cervix is only about four inches up, but lots of us don't think of finding out about it. But it's quite simple, it's a part of your body and actually belongs to you—not to the doctor! At the end of pregnancy it looks like a Victorian button cushion, plump and rounded, with the mucous plug like the button in the middle. When the cervix is really ready for labour to start it is said to be 'ripe'.

The teacher may want to say something about uterine action. It is easy to get tremendously involved about this subject, which is a very exciting one, to explain how, by using multiple intramyometrial microballoons, the contractile wave has been found to start in the cornual region, and to go on about 'triple descending gradients', asynchrony, tensile strength of the myometrium, and so on. Even though some of the husbands in particular will find this fascinating, I would not advise it. Although it is important to have read Caldeyro-Barcia, Friedman and others,* so that you can answer any further questions or know where to seek the answers, all information given in the antenatal class should be subordinate to the primary aim of helping a woman understand, and be able to work in harmony with, her own body.

So it is more relevant to the needs of expectant mothers to describe uterine action simply, at least at first, saying perhaps:

The uterus is the largest muscle in the human body, much larger than any muscle in a man's body—bigger even than the biceps of a champion boxer. It is not surprising that its activity when contracting can be overwhelming for someone unprepared for the hard work that it is going to do.

The first stage is the period during which the cervix is first being drawn up or 'effaced' and then opening wide, only instead of 'opening' we talk about 'dilatation'. The first labour contractions may be any number of minutes apart—as many as ten or fifteen, and often last about half or three-quarters of a minute. Gradually they come closer together, and rise higher at their peak, rather like waves of the sea following each other, or a great mountain range rising higher and higher. With each contraction the muscle fibres running from top to bottom of the uterus are shortened and thickened, and in time the upper part of the uterus becomes thick and the whole lower part is thinned out.

The wave of the contraction starts at the top of the uterus, and it has been suggested that there is something like a natural 'pacemaker' there which controls the waves, but the vast majority of women *feel* the contractions much lower down, at the front where the cervix is opening, in the small of the back, or all round from the cervix to the back, pulling like a tight, wide band of super-strong elastic.

When talking about the first stage you can help if you act the part

* On this subject the reading list I would advise for the teacher interested in this subject would include: Emanual A. Friedman, *Labor: Clinical Evaluation and Management* (New York, Appleton-Century-Crofts, 1967); the chapter on 'Factors Controlling the Action of the pregnant Human Uterus' by R. Caldeyro-Barcia in M. Knowlessor, ed., *Fifth Conference on Physiology of Prematurity* (New York, Josiah Macey Jr. Foundation, 1961); and the chapter on 'The Mechanism of Myometrial Function and Its Disorders', A. Csapo, in *Modern Trends in Obstetrics and Gynecology*, K. Bowes, ed. (London, Butterworth, 1955).

of the uterus, using your arms as if you were pulling up and shortening your whole body, with your legs acting as the cervix, bending and so shortening them first, and then gradually spreading your feet wider apart.

Many teachers dislike talking about forceps deliveries and shy away from the subject of 'complications'. With epidural anaesthesia outlet forceps are used so much as a matter of routine in many modern hospitals that it is important that the teacher should be able to discuss this without feeling uneasy, for example:

One of the ways in which the doctor can hurry delivery is to use forceps. They are two thin metal rods shaped rather like salad servers which hinge together. [Here it helps if you have some forceps in your hand with which to demonstrate, or use your hands, interlocking the thumbs.] They are used to cradle the baby's head, and are locked into position so that they cannot press in on the head. The doctor has to use a pull about as strong as that used to pull out a tight cork from a bottle of wine—long, firm and steady. Either local anaesthesia, like an injection at the dentist's, or epidural, or general anaesthesia may be used. If the mother is conscious she is able to cooperate to get the baby born.

A vacuum extractor is rather like a miniature vacuum cleaner, which is held against the baby's head (or buttocks) and draws it out by suction. The doctor can regulate the degree of suction used, and as with forceps deliveries nowadays too, the mother is usually asked to work *with* the doctor and her contractions.

With forceps there may be pressure marks on the head which go after a few days. With the vacuum extractor the baby may have a circular bump, in the area where the pressure was applied, for a few days.

Someone in the class will introduce *induction*, even if you do not; nowadays this frequently comes up in the first class:

The placenta has a limited life span—its own youth, maturity and old age. If tests of oestriol in the urine show that it is not working well labour may be induced for the sake of the baby, whose oxygen supply depends on the placenta functioning efficiently. Sometimes if a woman is ready to go into labour a large dose of castor oil (drop an effervescent vitamin c tablet and add a little gin and it does not taste so bad) is sufficient to start off contractions, or there is a pleasanter way—passionate love-making!

Often surgical induction, when the cervix is ripe, is an effective way of inducing labour, and the doctor sweeps the membranes, puncturing the bag of waters through the softened and slightly dilated cervix. (ARM means 'artificial rupture of the membranes'.) If this is insufficient to start off good labour contractions, or if the cervix is still hard, induction may take the form of an oxytocin drip; a hormone substance similar to that which naturally triggers off labour is dripped into a vein in the mother's arm to start contractions. At the same time a glucose drip gives the mother fresh energy. This may also be used if labour starts and then for some reason stops completely, or if labour is very long drawn out, and then it is called *accelerated labour*.

If you have your membranes ruptured your doctor may agree to let you wait four hours or so to see if labour will start spontaneously from that point, rather than inserting a drip immediately. If you start off under your own steam after the ARM you may never need a drip. So I think it is a good idea to discuss this with your doctor before the ARM.

There are many ways in which the teacher could talk about these subjects, and there is no correct formula. The important thing is that you should discover how you personally can express yourself most effectively. You will find that you are exploring the language of imagery and that the appropriate image becomes an essential tool of your vocabulary.

Teachers will evolve their own style of teaching if they create vivid imagery which is clear, with which they themselves feel comfortable, and which is designed to assist women in developing their own positive anticipatory fantasies of labour. To assess the value of exercises in preparation for childbirth is relatively easy, but not so easy to assess the value of anticipatory fantasies of this nature, largely because such fantasies are personal and intimate. My own impression from teaching many hundreds of mothers is that the woman who can fantasize, not only without anxiety but with pleasure, about her approaching labour is the one most likely to experience labour as a satisfying and pleasurable activity. The teacher's role in this can be constructive, supportive and understanding.

Somehow we have to learn how to convey to an expectant mother what labour feels like. This must always be done in terms of her own experience, proceeding from the known to the unknown, from that which is comprehended to that which is unfamiliar. To convey to primigravidae the physical and emotional sensations that accompany birth is difficult: we find it easier, perhaps, to transmit feelings associated with sight and sound rather than those associated with muscle tensions, pressure and the stretching of ligaments. The first rule is that one should never underestimate these sensations. In one English book on sexual adjustment, in which an attempt is made to define and describe orgasm, it is suggested that the nearest comparable physical sensation is that of a sneeze. While in the context of sexual adjustment that is merely funny, similar sorts of inadequate imagery used in reference to childbirth may produce trauma in the woman who is not sufficiently prepared to meet the powerful sensations of labour.

We have a problem similar to, but even more complicated than, that of a wine lover who is trying to convey the flavour of some particular wine. It is easy to be very imprecise; easy, also, to reduce it to the ludicrous.

The baby moves, and I discuss with them the sensations associated with this and with Braxton-Hicks contractions. Often one can learn a good deal about the mother's feelings concerning the baby when she interprets these sensations as unpleasant. The imagery in which other women describe their feelings is usefully shared with the group of expectant mothers. Remember that each woman has something from her own unique personal experience to teach us and it is up to us not only to teach but also to learn from her.

The woman teacher of preparation for childbirth who has also in the recent past borne children in full awareness is at a tremendous advantage if she can, at the same time, communicate her feelings. A man, however well informed, sympathetic and understanding, must be at a disadvantage. Every time I teach relaxation and contraction of the muscles of the abdominal wall and of the glutei I cannot help remembering the description given in one book for expectant mothers written by a male doctor in which contraction of these muscles was described as feeling 'as if one were wearing a pair of boy scout's shorts which were two sizes too small'. I think very few of his expectant mothers could ever have been in that situation. If he had described it in terms of pulling on wet jeans which were much too tight they might have understood rather better what he was talking about.

Uterine contractions are felt by many women to sweep towards them, rise in crescendo and then fade away like waves of the sea, so that wave imagery is very useful when describing the sensations they produce. This wave imagery is closely associated with the idea of rhythm, which is all important in harmonious psychosomatic adaptation to labour. One can explain how a woman must 'swim' over the wave and not allow it to envelop her, and to do this she needs go forward to meet it with her breathing instead of waiting until it is already on her. If she retreats from it it will almost certainly sweep over her. So she sets out to judge its size, and to keep on top of it with her breathing, adapting the rhythm and depth of her breathing to the curve of the wave. As it approaches its crest, her breathing is at its most light and rapid. Her breathing is always in relation, not to a chart on a wall or an illustration in a book, but to that particular contraction of her own uterus and to its rhythm and intensity. To change the image, it is as if the uterus were the conductor and she the orchestra; she learns to keep her eye on the conductor and respond immediately with the active relaxation and breathing that she has learned. With each wave of the sea the tide gradually flows farther in, bringing nearer the time when her baby will be in her arms. Sometimes the waves will get very rough; towards the end of the first stage they may seem to tower as high as a tidal wave, and then it is a little like bathing in a tempestuous sea, but it can be very exciting and wonderfully invigorating and refreshing. There are many possible extensions of this wave image; I have mentioned only a few.

In a way the childbirth educator needs to learn a new language. It is not just changing the statements in obstetric textbooks so that they are simple to understand. The challenge for each one of us is rather to use words creatively, to forge new phrases and images, so that the language of antenatal teaching becomes an art.

Discussion

Whatever the backgrounds of the mothers, in discussing emotional aspects of pregnancy the antenatal teacher's role is to open up discussion of subjects which group members may have felt were purely personal and to help them see that they are part of a common emotional experience. Expectant mothers usually greet with relief any information that other expectant mothers, too, have the same disturbed sleep or bad dreams, the same worries about the unborn child, or the same problems with in-laws.

A question designed to stimulate discussion, and one which is useful when couples attend classes together, is 'Do you want to bring up your child in the same way that you were brought up—or differently in any way?' Couples have often not really thought about this before as a problem to be solved, although many have been vaguely aware of it as a possible irritant. 'Do you feel these differences in approach might produce any friction in the early months after the baby is born?' 'Can we think of any ways in which a grandmother could be involved without your feeling that you are tripping over each other, or fighting over possession of the baby?' They can be encouraged to imagine how the 'replaced mother' may feel. Other expectant mothers will probably then express regret that their mothers, far from being too intrusive or demanding, are taking no interest at all in the coming baby. A few may have mothers overseas, and one or two may be bereaved. Discussion of this kind will help them all get their own relationships in perspective, see the advantages and disadvantages of their own situations, and what they can do about them in terms of their own practical and emotional preparation. Often a multipara will help with proposed solutions to conflict. One can go on from this discussion to talk about the roles of fathers in the family, and the way they see themselves in relation to their wives as mothers and to their children.

In a study of the modern urban family in the United States women[*] were asked, 'How is the relation between husband and wife changed by the presence of children?' In the context of the antenatal class, this question would be better preceded by two others: Do you think there are changes in the relation between husband and wife when a baby is on the way? *and* And what about after the baby is born . . . any changes do you think? In this discussion the teacher will have in mind certain main types of change which occur as the result

[*] Helen Lopata, *Occupation: Housewife* (New York, OUP Paperback, 1972).

of childbearing, and is ready to describe some of these changes if they are not perceived as important by group members.

In conclusion, let us consider some other questions which may initiate discussion and which, used with discretion and with suitable changes of phrase, can help group members think about emotional aspects of the experience of childbearing in a mutually rewarding way:

Do you remember how you felt when you learned you were pregnant? What came into your mind?

What differences were there between your feelings then and the way you feel now about the pregnancy and the baby?

The first three months of pregnancy; can you think back to them? Were there any physical problems like tiredness or nausea or anything like that? And how did you feel about being pregnant and the changes that were happening in you? Do you think your husband felt in any way the same or differently? Was it easy to talk about the coming baby so he would understand?

What do you think ideal grandparents are like?

Do you feel you've learned anything special about being a mother from your own mother? And the men, from your own fathers?

Do you think you'll be very like your own mother/father, or different in any way?

Did you feel any differently about pregnancy once the first three months were up?

Can you remember how you felt when you first noticed the baby's movements? What did they feel like? And now? Do you find it a pleasant or disturbing sensation?

Do you have any worries about the baby at all—its safety or its being normal?

Do you wonder whether you'll make a good mother? Do you think good mothers are born or made?

And what about good fathers; are they born or made?

How do you feel during these last three months? Weary, or impatient, or, how many women feel, that they are turning into a vegetable?

How are you sleeping? Do you dream? Do you find you get very vivid dreams, or bad dreams? Perhaps you find you worry in the middle of the night? What sort of thing do you worry about then?

Do you like going to the antenatal clinic, or is there anything about it you dislike?

Do you feel that you already know the baby inside you, perhaps even its sex, or do you feel that it is a real stranger? Do you find yourself wanting a boy or a girl particularly?

Do you have daydreams about the baby? What sort?

Have you talked much about being together in labour? Do you like the idea? Or perhaps you have rather different attitudes?

We all tense up at one time or another. Can you think of anything in the last week that has made you go tense? What kinds of situation do you think makes you contract muscles unnecessarily?

Do you ever wonder whether you'll be able to love your baby? Do you think it will be easy to be fond of it, or not?

Is this what you saw happening in your life, say, four years ago? . . .

Is this what you wanted to be doing now?

Those of you who have recently given up jobs, did you find the change from going out to work and being at home all day at all difficult?

6

The Psychology of Pregnancy

The pregnant woman experiences a startling transformation in her body, a change even more dramatic than that of growing from a girl into a woman, and one much more marked than anything a man experiences. Although childbirth education classes usually teach breathing and relaxation, they can also provide a valuable opportunity for women to discuss their changing bodies and the emotional effects of pregnancy.

The Normal Psychological Stresses of Pregnancy

Psychiatric literature treats the body images characteristic of pregnancy as if they were symptoms of neurosis and were all pathological. But it is clear from discussions in antenatal classes that nearly *every* woman experiences profound and far-reaching psychic changes including modifications in her fantasies about her body boundaries and her internal geography. This is nothing to do with neurosis. It is a normal process of adaptation to the demands of pregnancy.

No expectant mother can exist on exactly the same terms with her body as before the pregnancy. She is taken over and weighed down by another life, which inhabits her every moment of every day and night.

Most women discover that they run through a wide range of emotions about the pregnancy at different stages. They frequently found acceptance difficult in the first three months, when the physio-logical adjustments necessary often caused tiredness before the pregnancy had reached the stage when people give them extra con-sideration. It is in early pregnancy that the woman may feel, in the words of one pregnant antenatal teacher, 'like a ship on a stormy sea, out of balance, seeking a new equilibrium in the waves of physical change'.

Some time between the fourth and sixth month, the other being in utero asserts itself—knocks, squirms and bounces—and as preg-nancy advances proclaims its presence in no uncertain way. 'Her pregnancy begins to act like a magnet, drawing her thoughts more and more inside herself.' There is a two-way conversation: one with people around her and the world outside and one with her inner world. For the most part women feel that they adjust with ease in the second trimester, enjoying the novelty of pregnancy, the extra attention, and the increasing awareness of another life existing inside them.

There are times when the woman forgets her pregnancy, but then she is overwhelmed by its reality as she catches sight of herself in a shop window, perhaps, a strange and enormous figure like, as one ex-Playboy Bunny put it, 'an enormous hippo wallowing in the mud', or when the fetus kicks her awake in the night. Sometimes expectant mothers enjoy these reminders of pregnancy, but they are often unpleasant, arising from what are called in obstetric books 'minor discomforts of pregnancy', which, in fact, can be uncomfortable in the extreme: indigestion, heartburn, itching, heavy perspiration, backache, cramp and varicose veins—to name but a few.

Approximately two-thirds of the number of women attending antenatal classes say that they become weary, apprehensive and have interrupted sleep in the last trimester, sometimes with intermittent depression and disturbing fantasies concerning both themselves and the baby. In the last three months there are times when the expectant mother feels that she has become merely a container for a developing fetus. One woman said, 'I am being used. My body is being used, and I can't do anything about it.'

In many ways this is an accurate assessment of her physical condi-tion. The weight gain alone, of between 9 kg (20 lbs) and 12·7 kg

(28 lbs)—about 25 per cent of her nonpregnant weight—3·2 kg (7 lbs) or more of baby, 72 g (24 oz) of placenta, 91 g (2 lbs) of amniotic fluid, 136 g (3 lbs) or more additional weight in the breasts and uterine wall, 5·4 kg (12 lbs) increase in maternal body fluids, and perhaps 4·5 kg (10 lbs) of extra fat stored under the skin around hips and buttocks and across her back) would be enough to make her feel that her body had been invaded and taken over.

Other remarkable physical changes are occurring too. There are profound respiratory modifications; with an increased tidal volume of air, the woman's oxygen consumption is raised by approximately 20 per cent, and her lower ribs flare out as the uterus rises and presses against them. There is extra protein storage in the liver. The heart gets larger and has to work harder as the blood flow increases. The woman's raised metabolism means that she gets hot and sticky, and feels she is carrying around her own central heating mechanism— one which cannot be turned off, even when there is a heat wave. The enlarged uterus presses on the veins of the lower half of her body and may produce varicose veins of her vulva and legs, and haemorrhoids. A reduction of gastric secretions can result in nausea, and partial relaxation of sphincters in her gastrointestinal tract may lead to heartburn.

In fact there is a lot happening, quite apart from a growing fetus. Her whole body serves the needs of the child which is to be born. It also becomes alien, no longer the friendly well-known body with familiar dimensions, but one that is changing from week to week.

Between six and four weeks before the expected date of delivery the expectant mother often experiences a sudden failure of nerve, focused either on the labour or on the formidable task of being a good-enough mother. This emerged in a conversation between Sarah and Tom when she announced: 'Tom does not want to be at the birth.' I asked, 'Why not?' and she replied, 'Because of the blood.' Tom said, 'No, it's not blood.' She turned to him and said aggressively, 'You wouldn't want to see a road accident!' Tom replied, 'I am desperately disappointed that she doesn't want me there', and at last Sarah could say quite simply, 'I am awfully scared!' Another couple were discussing breastfeeding, and she said,

'He has always advocated breastfeeding. It is a passion of his', and then added, 'He would make a much better mother than me!' expressing her real anxiety about meeting the challenge of motherhood.

This is a crisis period, when the pregnant woman is like an actress before the curtain goes up on the opening night, when she fears that she will forget all she has learned and worries that she has been over-confident. It is, in one woman's words

an abrupt breakthrough of cold reality. It is like living in a warm, cosily lit house where a door is blown open on to the dark night outside. Suddenly the bump is a *baby*—a baby which, somehow, some day, has to get born. Whether by the birth canal or a Caesarean, whether it lives or dies, it is *in* and must come *out*.

For each woman pregnancy has its private meaning. Only when she lies awake in the night may fantasies be dredged up from the deeper levels of the mind which do not normally impinge on her rational thoughts. Approximately half the number of women attending classes reported that at some stage of pregnancy they lay awake in the night thinking. Sometimes, too, in the images occurring in dreams the pregnant woman catches a glimpse of feelings about her body, her pregnancy and the baby which she did not know she had. Such a woman has a capacity for reflection which not all expectant mothers have, and perhaps for the majority pregnancy unfolds with the inner meanings on the other side of a screen, as it were, while the woman continues to live 'as normal' and adopts the socially correct attitudes about the coming baby. This is an opportunity lost for supportive psychotherapy in a *normal life crisis*.

The pregnancy is also part of a relationship between a man and woman, and *he* has to live with it too. He may wonder why his wife weeps sometimes for no reason at all, is affronted at a chance remark or a joke he made about her figure, why she cannot face meeting her mother-in-law or has a row with her mother, gets sentimental over baby clothes, laughs uproariously at an incident which is not all that funny, becomes depressed about world politics, or reacts emotionally to minor occurrences which formerly she would hardly have noticed. He may shrug his shoulders and think Oh, women! This attitude is taken by his wife as a reflection on her value and evidence that he does not love her. He may look it up in the books and is told, 'Pregnant women are vulnerable', but unless he can understand more than this his tendency is to escape to the office, the arms of another woman, back to his mother, or into his books. Instead of drawing them closer together in a shared experience the pregnancy then pulls them apart and creates what can become a permanent rift in their marriage. Here again, the childbirth preparation group can help their mutual understanding and sharing.

Sometimes the pattern of emotional change in pregnancy is very different, and the woman does not react to it at first because she only half believes in it and, as several women in the classes put it, 'feels a fraud'. The first recognized fetal movements produce a shocked reaction in which she sees the baby as an invader of her body and a threat to her identity. As time passes she comes to terms with it, but may meet a new challenge with the birth and the confrontation with the baby as a separate being outside her body.

Because a woman is happy in her pregnancy we should never take it for granted that she will adjust easily to motherhood and all that it entails. Pregnancy is part of a continuum, and although for some women it brings deep content, new stresses come once the baby is born.

Emotional Crises in Pregnancy and After

Not many women have mental breakdowns during pregnancy. It is, in fact, a time of extraordinary pliability. The real conflicts come afterwards. Responsible care of the childbearing woman does not end with labour, or even with the postnatal check-up, but recognizes that the birth is but one crisis in a continuing psychosexual process and that after the baby is born women are living through some of the experiences for which they should have been prepared during pregnancy. In teaching or counselling the woman with a baby in utero the antenatal teacher, the obstetrician and midwife need always to remain aware that she is going to have a baby outside in her arms and have to relate herself to it, not so very far ahead. The quality of that relationship may depend to a large extent on the kind of emotional support that she is offered during pregnancy.

There are women who use a pregnancy to serve their own neurotic needs. For some the whole of pregnancy means *possession*, and they feel that they have at last locked the proof of love inside them. In Freudian terms the pregnancy symbolizes the prolongation of coitus. These mothers may hold on to the pregnancy, and later to the baby, with satisfied but underlying anxious pride of ownership. Some expectant mothers are so in-turned and fearful for the baby during pregnancy that they not only refuse to have intercourse but do not feel able to relate to their husbands physically at all, so that there is little or no sexual pleasuring of any kind. Although such a woman enjoys her pregnancy, she may feel lost and empty once the pregnancy is over and she can no longer hold the baby inside her. And although at first she can hold the baby tightly in her arms, she is unable to cope with the child's movements of exploration and independence away from her and encounters special stresses when the baby becomes a toddler who rebels and has tantrums. Here again, pregnancy contentment is not really a sign that all is well, but is a precursor of subsequent emotional turmoil.

Sometimes pregnancy is eagerly grasped as a practical solution to the problem of holding on to love which threatens to go, and of desperately trying to mend a marriage ('a child will bring us closer together') or even of replacing a love which has obviously disappeared. Couples who have a baby to mend a marriage are heading for disaster. The introduction of a new and demanding member into the family can break rather than make the relationship.

Pregnancy as possession may be a matter of creating another being from whom to claim love. The baby then becomes a doll to be played with. This woman, too, may be very happy in her pregnancy, but faces problems if the infant is not a 'cuddly' baby, proves unresponsive or irritable, or takes attention and affection from herself. One mother said of her two year old, 'I gave up so much for Judith, and I have had nothing back from her. She has given me nothing at all.' The offer of affection is a currency to gain the security of being loved. These mothers may also be terribly disappointed at the real baby which is put in their arms when compared with the fantasy baby of pregnancy. It is a boy when they were sure they were going to have a girl, or vice versa. They may even feel it cannot be theirs. They romanticize the appearance of a newborn child and are unable to tolerate any slight deviation from the perfect either in physical appearance or behaviour. Some of these babies will be those at special risk of maternal rejection or hostility or emotional withdrawal. The antenatal teacher is probably in a unique position for seeing which women need special care and understanding if they are to grow into adequate mothers.

Pregnancy may be used as a means of retreat from effort. For some women, who have not met the standards their parents set for them, pregnancy is the only achievement in their lives. They may have failed academic examinations or for some reason have not attained parent-set goals. They feel failures, and the only thing they can do is to make a baby. One woman said, for example, 'This is the first thing I have done which my parents haven't wanted and planned for me. Mother would like to take over. But I am going to have my baby *my* way!' The pregnancy is then an expression of adolescent crisis, and if used constructively can point the way out of it and be a means of growing up.

For some very lonely women pregnancy means that they are no longer solitary. Male/female roles in our society are still such that there are many marriages where the husband goes off to work leaving his wife in their charming suburban dwelling aching with loneliness and boredom. One woman who found that she and her husband were inhabiting two different social worlds, said: 'When you have a baby inside you you are not alone any more.' For other women who have an unrealistic dread of isolation or of being dissolved as personalities and losing their identity too, pregnancy may bring a new stability and contentment (and this is particularly true of the agoraphobic who may be able to face going out for the first time when she feels fetal movements) but with the birth they lose the baby in its special intrauterine relationship with them. Delivery then may initiate a phase of stress as they try to adjust to the situation of a baby outside who is no longer part of them. Unless given emotional support then they are totally bereft and lost. This adjustment entails grieving, when they mourn the fantasy baby they have lost and accept the real baby.

Some women express overt aggression against the male in pregnancy. Here again, pregnancy can bring a short-lived satisfaction. In my own classes I had four unmarried women who rejected their men once they had achieved impregnation and were determined that the pregnancy, birth and the baby itself should be their own work, and not shared with a man. Only when they met the fathers in classes who were supporting and helping their wives did they begin to see that it might be good, after all, to share the process of child-bearing with the father, and in some cases the unmarried fathers also came to learn how they could help and took on their share of responsibility and caring.

To other women pregnancy is a humiliation and provides opportunities for masochistic satisfaction. Feelings of degradation and shame during pregnancy are associated with ideas about dirt and cleanliness and evil and good, in which sex may be seen as disgusting, and in which negative attitudes to defecation, intercourse and child-bearing are inextricably mingled. One woman said, 'He uses me like a lavatory and then I find I'm pregnant.' In certain Mediterranean societies this is a culturally approved reaction to pregnancy, and one in which the individual woman's values about pregnancy and birth, and her behaviour, reflect the dominant cultural motif. Within our own society it suggests emotional disturbance.

Some women feel invaded by a hostile and alien organism. Pregnancy is a sickness of which the woman is ashamed and which she fights to keep under control to continue as normal. One woman said, 'I hate my thickening waist and oozing body. I feel disgusted when I look in a mirror. Just a white, pulpy mess. The baby is like a cancer which goes on growing and draws life from me, whatever I do.' Each movement of the baby may be experienced as an act of aggression. 'The baby waits till I am lying down and then he really fights me.' Such women may engage desperately in the expulsive stage of labour with complete lack of coordination. There is a terrible urgency about getting rid of the baby, and they push it out as if they were forcing poison out of their bodies.

These varying attitudes tend to be associated with attitudes towards breast or bottle feeding. When the mother thought of the baby in utero as a cancer, for instance, and the swollen, milky breast also as an ugly growth, lactation is approached with distaste. On the other hand, women who seek to maintain the intrauterine relationship as long as possible, because of their own emotional needs, may approach breastfeeding with very positive feelings and continue it well into the second or the third year of life, not because the baby needs the milk, or even the comfort of sucking, but because *they* need the baby.

These are just some of the feelings that women can have about their pregnancies, and many of them overlap. When one considers the enormous changes that occur during forty weeks, it is remarkable how many women make the adjustment smoothly. In concentrating attention on difficulties and failures of adjustment I do not wish to suggest that many women do not thoroughly enjoy their pregnancies, and experience them as a time of radiant well-being and joy. The majority of expectant mothers in my classes think of bearing a child in terms of fruition, and see pregnancy as a process of emotional and physiological fulfilment. In many cases the husbands share this attitude, and, in discussion they say, 'I like the lovely ripe curve of your tummy', 'I love pregnant ladies', or 'I think it's a gorgeous shape!'

Pregnancy in Other Societies

In some ways the physical and social changes of pregnancy are comparable to those of adolescence. It is a phase of recurrent, but normal, crises. Whereas 'modern' society recognizes the problems of adolescence, it is much less aware of those of pregnancy, and women are left without emotional support in the process of maturation through childbearing. This is in marked contrast to primitive and peasant communities, in which, as we shall see later, transitional rituals define the pregnant woman's role as she passes over 'the bridge' into motherhood, older women teach her appropriate behaviour and attitudes, and where, to a much greater degree than in modern society, members of the peer group of other mothers share with her the experience through which she is passing.

When women talk about the changes involved in pregnancy, it emerges that it is a common experience for expectant mothers in industrialized, urban society to be alone, cut off from previous social and work contacts, in late pregnancy, in a way that they have never been before. They become social isolates. Many say that although at first they loved giving up work and being free of office routines, for instance, they soon began to miss their colleagues and being part of a work team. This abrupt shift of role from being economically productive to being a mother does not occur in peasant societies, and neither the rhythms of work nor the patterns of social relationships are much disturbed by pregnancy. Moreover, the pregnancy is far from being a solitary experience, or one which only has meaning for the couple. It is recognized and acclaimed as significant not only for the marriage, which is often only recognized as complete when the first child comes, but for the kinship group to which the expectant mother belongs, the descent group into which the baby is being born, and the larger society.

The taboos and restrictions on behaviour characteristic of pregnancy in these societies, which survive for expectant mothers in modern society only as old wives' tales, reflect the concern of the whole community, and although they seem mere superstitions, they fill functions which the modern system of antenatal care may fail to perform.

Dietary prohibitions and regulations, sympathetic magic, physical actions bearing on the woman's sense of her own body, and rules which draw in the father of the child and involve him, too, in the preparation for the baby combine to make the pregnancy a socially controlled process in which each member of the family into which the child is born has his or her correct part to play.

The *couvade*, in which the father takes on part of the pregnancy, labour or lying-in, bearing it for his wife, is an expression of the same paternal responsibilities, and an indication that the woman is supported by a man who shares responsibility for the outcome of parturition. Although the couvade in its most dramatic form, when the husband goes to bed and labours 'for' the woman while she continues her work to the time of delivery, has attracted most attention, it is by no means its most common expression. More frequent is the 'lying-in' of the husband after childbirth, and still more common is the assumption by the man of various pregnancy symptoms and discomforts, as well as antenatal regulations and taboos. The couvade syndrome is also well known in the West, where it is not unusual for a prospective father to suffer backache, toothache, stomach ache or nausea. I interviewed one country-woman in Oxfordshire who had lost her baby in the fourth month of pregnancy. Her husband had been having backache from the time when he realized his wife was pregnant. He continued to suffer until the day when the baby would have been due if the pregnancy had continued, and then experienced a very bad bout of backache, after which it disappeared completely. His sister commented: 'He carried for Jenny.' In the United States a similar case occurred in which a woman said of her husband, who vomited every morning during six pregnancies, 'My man he allus does my pukin' for me.'*

In some societies the pregnant woman is helped to relate to the baby in utero, not simply as 'a bump' but as a person, by making a doll which represents the spirit of the coming child. Among the Mansi tribes of Siberia† she makes one no bigger than her thumb out of dried brown growth of the birch tree. This doll is consecrated, decorated and kept in her sewing bag. Every now and again she must take it out and kiss it, and from the way in which it swings when suspended from its ribbons women can foretell whether the birth will be easy and the child healthy. Three months after the birth it is burned, and its ashes mixed with water in which the mother bathes herself and her child. Thereby her spirit child becomes her real child. The doll fulfils the dual purpose of helping the mother to focus on the idea of the coming child and later to relate the baby to which she has actually given birth to the fantasy child of pregnancy. One important function shared by pregnancy dream prophecies—common in many societies—and by the spirit doll is that an emotional continuity between the pregnancy and the weeks after

* Vance Randolph, *Ozark Superstitions* (New York, Columbia University Press, 1947).

† E. I. Rombandeeva, 'Some Observances and Customs of the Mansi (Voguls) in Connection with Childbirth', *Popular Beliefs and Folklore Traditions in Siberia*, V. Dioszeg, ed. (Bloomington, Indiana Univ. Press, 1960).

birth is established by a socially recognized and culturally patterned act.

In traditional societies the mother's behaviour and thinking in pregnancy and birth are also interwoven with the religious system. The months of waiting and the labour and delivery are not clinical conditions, but *ritual states.*

There is an Egyptian hymn to Aton which expresses the religious significance of parturition:

> Creator of seed in women,
> Thou who makest fluid into man,
> Who maintainest the son in the womb of his mother,
> Who soothest him with that which stills his weeping,
> Thou nurse even in the womb,
> Who givest breath to sustain all that he has made!
> When he descends from the womb to breathe
> On the day when he is born,
> Thou openest his mouth completely,
> Thou suppliest his necessities.*

It is an affirmation of the deeper significance of birth which is almost wholly missing in our own society. In the absence of values about birth which are openly stated and held in common in society, the parturient woman is left primarily as a patient enduring her pregnancy as a disorder or sickness.

In the West, many a pregnant woman feels as if she is treated as a childbearing mechanism, the efficiency of which must be regulated by correct antenatal treatment and obstetric routines, rather than as a person. This may be done with the same impersonality with which a car is serviced. As the woman lies, her lower end bare, on a hard examination table, with her legs up in stirrups, and the doctor prods, surrounded by a group of students, she may feel, 'This is *my* body! It belongs to me, not you'. One subject that comes up for discussion in each course of classes, sometimes frequently, is anxiety about hospital procedures. Of ninety-five expectant mothers taught

* Translated by John A. Wilson; James B. Pritchard, ed., *Ancient Near Eastern Texts Relating to the Old Testament,* 2nd ed. (Princeton, N.J., Princeton University Press, 1955).

in the year 1974, eighty-seven of the women reported some incident which had produced anxiety, frustration or hostility, and many experienced repeated situations in which they felt unable to communicate with doctors or midwives.

Little of this may be perceived by the doctor, who may believe that the occasional lighthearted joke is sufficient to keep most of his patients placid and sensible. Yet when I asked groups of expectant mothers Do you like going to the hospital antenatal clinic? *and* Do you get a chance to talk and ask questions? discussion invariably followed in which one woman after another told of her distress after attending the clinic. The antenatal clinic visit to a large modern hospital, entailing being 'processed' and often examined by strangers, is often seen by expectant mothers as an ordeal to be endured.

Women frequently see induction of labour, particularly when an oxytocin drip is used to initiate and control contractions, as the final point in this taking over of their bodies. Only two of the women in my series (admittedly a self-selected group of women, for the most part middle class, who sought out antenatal preparation) did not express apprehension about induction and 'active management' and some became distressed, as did one woman who, according to her husband, 'wept all night' before being admitted for induction. It seems that implied in the need for induction of labour is a reproductive inadequacy and unworthiness, which can strike at self-esteem and the sense of the body as good.

In peasant societies recognized psychic changes in pregnancy are catered for by facilitating rituals and specific institutionalized ways of scrutinizing psychic phenomena, such as dream analysis and the recounting of myth. These rites and practices floodlight the transitional state of pregnancy and also circumscribe and frame it so that it is seen as of special significance. The taboos, prohibitions and regulations of diet and behaviour imply that pregnancy is a difficult time, that the mother is treading on unsure ground and must be observant about what she is doing. They are stating, in effect, that you have to 'grow a baby' carefully. Because the rites involve the participation of others in the community, they also imply that the changes through which the expectant mother is passing are important not only for her as an individual but for the larger society.

Compared with this, in the more developed societies, the culture of pregnancy, although technologically superior, is ritually impoverished. One cannot go back to the traditions of a peasant society, but perhaps one ought to remember that pregnancy can be not only a waiting time but a growing time. Given good emotional support and education for parenthood, it can be a time of preparation not only for the birth of a child but for the birth of a woman as a mother and a man as a father.

7

Mothers, Daughters and Teachers

The relationship between a pregnant woman and her own mother is a major theme in the way in which she becomes a mother herself. Overdependence upon the mother, for example, whether it takes the form of leaning on her and trying to win her approval or that of a violent ambivalence (in which the mother's importance may be often denied, but in which she is, nevertheless, the central figure in a woman's life) not only can make it difficult for her to achieve the independence and self-control which is necessary for a happy labour but can make her adjustment to motherhood and its responsibilities and decisions almost impossible. One of our own responsibilities may be to help a girl grow up during her pregnancy, and to become a mature woman, capable of deciding her own course of action.

The relationship between the antenatal teacher and the pupils is not static, but dynamic, and as with all close therapeutic relationships of this kind, the pupil frequently passes through a phase of positive transference. The infantile expectant mother, in particular, may ring up frequently, bring her friends and relations, and be enthusiastic about 'the method'. At some stage she may also go through a corresponding phase of negative transference, expressed, perhaps, in the form of feeling 'let down' by the teacher, absence from or late arrival at classes, and the deliberate introduction of negative material into the discussion. Most teachers welcome the positive transference—it gives them a feeling of confidence and success—but find it difficult to tolerate the negative.

Both the adoration and the pulling away can be part of a developing relationship in which the pupil is outgrowing her need for enthusiastic discipleship and is beginning to find her own feet, and it is up to the teacher to see that it is used in this way. I remember feeling first irritation, but then relief as I was told that a disturbed and anxious woman who had been very dependent on me in a difficult labour in which her baby's life was at stake and during which I had had to work extremely hard, had said afterwards, 'Oh, I knew it would be all right. The holy angels were all around my bed.' Dependence on the holy angels is preferable to overdependence on me, and it is part of our task as teachers to wean the pupils away from us and help them to grow up.

The problem of overdependence upon the teacher is a real one, because those women who are still overdependent on their mothers seek maternal support in this crisis of their lives and lean on a teacher as a wise, powerful and loving mother figure. Unfortunately some teachers willingly and eagerly assume this role (which answers a deep-seated need for power or for love in their own psyches), play it up and exploit it, and make their pupils even more dependent than they need to be. Authoritarian, compelling, the teacher stands before her class: her every word initiates immediate, unquestioning, correct response. 'Breathe in' she commands. And they all breathe in. 'And OUT', and they all breathe out. This instantaneous obedience, this utter dependence, is unhealthy for both teacher and taught. The pupils are well-drilled, confident, but their self-assurance is deceptive, and in emotionally unstable or immature women it is a firmness 'analogous to that which a corset provides for an individual whose backbone is injured'*—useful in an emergency, but of no permanent value. A discipline merely imposed from without will do nothing except, possibly, tide a woman over the actual crisis of labour. Somehow the teacher has to help each pupil find a centre of gravity within herself.

* Karen Horney, *New Ways in Psychoanalysis*, 4th ed. (London, Routledge, 1961.)

The Infantile Primipara

The mother–daughter relationship often has a primary impact on the process of childbearing, particularly in the case of overdependent and emotionally immature girls having their first baby. These expectant mothers are sufficiently frequently met with by those teaching preparation for childbirth to form a category of their own, already studied by de Senarclens and Picot in Switzerland. No teacher can afford to neglect the strength of the mother–daughter relationship when preparing these pupils. We must help the pregnant girl to make ventures in independence, or at the very least to transfer her dependence from the mother to the husband. In those marriages I have observed where the girl's mother has been dominant and really the main power figure in an emotional triangle, the stress of pregnancy, birth and early motherhood has inevitably been great.

A girl who is still clinging to her mother in infantile dependence is likely to find labour a shattering experience. She leans on the teacher, refusing to do anything for herself, wanting all instruction to be very simple and the guidelines definite, and seeking authoritarian statements and control. Some teachers, by their very nature, more readily offer this and use a more mechanical and rigid form of instruction and didactic classroom techniques.

The techniques of psychoprophylaxis can be taught in this way, leaving little choice to the labouring woman, so that no decision-making is necessary. She follows a prescribed mechanical technique, obeys instructions implicitly, and trusts her teacher rather than her own body. Results, in performance in childbirth (which is and must be the immediate aim), are quickly achieved under these conditions; but there is danger that in avoiding the basic emotional problems of overdependence on the mother, or on other women who fit the mother image, the newly delivered girl is launched on motherhood utterly unprepared for its responsibilities, the necessary decision-making associated with infant care and, in urban communities, for the social isolation of the middle-class mother tied to the house and to young children.

To replace the mother with a strong mother-figure in the form of an antenatal teacher, who may even be willing to assist the girl also during her labour, is merely to circumvent this problem and to delay its possible solution. Pregnancy, bringing with it a new image of the self, involves the sort of emotional crisis which can lead to the eventual solution of this problem of overdependence. Pregnancy is a magnificent opportunity of growing up emotionally which it is a sheer waste not to seize.

The difficulties in both childbirth and early motherhood which these infantile primiparae are likely to encounter are predictable. In pregnancy the girl guards her child in utero a little like a doll. She may be late to recognize its movements—not until after the twentieth week—and when they occur strongly in late pregnancy she may be very disturbed by them. She is surprised at the child's animation and strength and may feel that its kicking is a sign of aggression against her. But she often quite enjoys pregnancy and the amount of attention this brings, and while the child is still in utero, requiring nothing of her, she maintains an emotional equilibrium. She becomes very distressed if she finds that the breathing or posture she has been taught in classes is not approved of by the midwife or obstetrician. She is anxious to conform and is usually an obedient patient. After the birth the new mother who is still in infantile dependence on her own mother tends to be bewildered by the baby, to be unable to react maternally (that is, within the context of the cultural patterning of maternity in modern society), and to be troubled by the inability to cope. She tries desperately to please the baby in the same way that she strives anxiously to please her mother. *But* the baby cries. This seems to constitute the preliminary condition for the development of one sort of depression following childbirth.

In these cases depression is predictable during pregnancy, and it is important that the teacher remembers that simply giving these women what they so patently desire—motherly sympathy, firm training and an unalterable doctrine— evades the real issue, and thus predisposes them to depression following childbirth.

The understanding midwife or health visitor encounters mild postpartum depression frequently not only in the immediate postpartum days but at any time in the first few weeks following birth. Its incidence does not always find a place in clinical records because it is expected and usually considered commonplace. It is only when it does not seem to be getting any better, when the young mother is discovered again and again collapsed in tears, when her husband fails to improve the condition with his reiterated advice to 'snap out of it', that further advice is sought and the family doctor consulted. It is often then explained in terms of the unbalanced endocrine system.

In one sense, of course, all women with first babies are unprepared for the responsibilities of motherhood in our society. Girl children are given little or no preparation, except through doll play, for motherhood. And even their dolls may be babies no longer, but teenagers with jutting breasts and elaborately back-combed hair styles. Girl children share very little in our modern two- or three-child family in the care of younger siblings, and it is accepted that baby care is limited to the mother of the child, much of it taking place in relative privacy. It is rare to see a mother breastfeeding her child in public.

Women in our society are more or less insulated from baby care until they are confronted with their offspring. But many quickly adapt themselves. The infantile primipara is faced with a more severe handicap. The doll baby in utero is very different from the real child crying in its cot. It was automatically nourished and cared for in her body, but now she must do something about it to keep it alive. Although parenting classes may help, they do not solve the problem of her basic emotional overdependence. Her mother is often ready to rush in to care for the new baby and to give advice, thus increasing the daughter's belief in her own inability to care for her child. When the baby cries she is alerted by its signals, but unable to act constructively or meaningfully. She cannot identify herself with her mother and thus feed the child and soothe it, but behaves as if she herself were the baby needing care and love. Her self-pity can easily prove irritating and exhausting to those who most want to help her.

A Case History in a Nutshell

One woman was sent to me by her doctor because of a traumatic first labour followed by severe depression and threatened depression in the first month of her second, unwanted pregnancy. She suffered from an exaggerated dependence upon her mother, who lived in the next village and to whom she had written every day of her life since her marriage, except at weekends when they visited each other.

When I first saw her she was threatening suicide. Her husband stayed home from work and did all the housework and cooking and cared for the child whom they described as a 'problem'; his wife sat and stared at the wall, with fits of weeping. She started to talk about her mother whom she described as 'a worrier like me' and 'possessive'. It soon emerged that the two women were involved in conflict over possession of the child, and the younger one felt guilty over her lack of control over the little boy. She lived next door to a woman with a baby who woke and cried at night. The walls were thin and every night this happened she relived in terror her own infantile dependence. 'I go tense. I cannot sleep. I am almost out of my mind.' She could not tolerate a crying baby and, when her own small child cried, panicked and was unable to do anything for him.

The husband himself was imprisoned in a relationship from which escape seemed equally difficult. His mother had been an invalid since his adolescence, and he had been her chief nurse. He confessed to us both, weeping, that he had married hoping to get away from it all, only to find that his wife was demanding the same services from him. For most of the five years since the birth of the first child she had refused her husband intercourse because of her fear of conceiving. 'It's a wonder he hasn't left me,' she said, in a moment of sudden sympathy. He began to realize that in going from one invalid to another he had derived emotional satisfaction from being needed, as a nurse, rather than a husband. So he had been colluding with his wife in her illness.

They started to discuss their problems together in private consultation, and it helped that he saw that it was not just *her* problem. After a while she turned to me and said that her mother had become ill in order to claim her love. From the time of that interview she no longer wrote her mother every day. By the last trimester of pregnancy she was much more cheerful and was a very eager member of the class. She said that she had decided to have her baby *her* way; after all it was her child and not her mother's, and the husband and wife, in doing exercises together, and in feeling more able to discuss their difficulties, shared a new understanding. In the weeks prior to the expected date of delivery she had a crisis of fear, and hypertension. She was very disturbed and particularly feared that she might get postnatal depression again. She also had a horror of being left alone in labour, as she was the time before (in hospital), and of the stretching preceding the birth of the baby's head, but responded well to reassurance.

A domiciliary confinement was agreed upon. Posterior at the onset of labour, the baby rotated spontaneously to the anterior. No sedation or analgesics were necessary, in spite of the anterior lip which delayed the onset of the second stage. She found control of her breathing and relaxation easy throughout her labour. Her husband, who had earlier in her pregnancy not wanted to be present, helped her, sponging her face, massaging her as he had been taught and encouraging her. Her control at delivery was excellent and the sensations she described as pleasant. Her attendants remarked upon her cooperation, and she herself felt that much was due to her husband's presence and assistance, which she felt was essential. She described her whole labour as marvellous both at the time and afterwards. Six weeks after the birth she was breastfeeding with great success (she had not been able to feed the first baby) and said she was enjoying the child in a way she had never been able to with the first one. Although she faced problems afterwards she seemed much better able to verbalize them, and severe depression did not recur.

This is but one rather spectacular example of a woman who was unable to mature in relation to her husband and to her child because of infantile dependence on a possessive mother.

From one point of view—admittedly a very one-sided one—every girl usurps her mother's role when she marries and has children. Occasionally the older woman, especially if she is widowed—if her own marriage has been rather a failure and she feels unwanted and unloved—resents the younger one and is openly jealous of her, but fortunately this is the exception rather than the rule.

Even so, some women feel almost guilty about having babies, as if pregnancy were a right they had insufficient maturity to claim, somehow as if they were taking them away from their own mothers.

Where a woman in a happy love relationship with a man unconsciously feels that she can take as it were the place that her mother took with her husband and now gains satisfactions that her mother enjoyed and that she as a child was denied, then she is able to feel equal to her mother, and to enjoy the same happiness, rights and privileges as her mother did, but without injuring and robbing her.*

With young couples who are able to adjust easily to parenthood they are in fact 'happily recreating their own early family lives'.

Often during pregnancy a woman feels closely drawn towards her mother, and occasionally a mother who is unhappy or lonely takes advantage of this and, without realizing that she is doing so, may come between husband and wife and make the husband feel isolated and unwanted.

Understandably a woman pregnant for the first time would want to learn from her own mother's experience, but it is vitally important for the marriage that the husband should know that he is needed, that he can help his wife through her pregnancy and also actually in labour, if he wishes.

The teacher should be particularly alert to possible emotional problems of this kind when a mother turns up with her daughter for a private interview or lesson. The mother should be gently persuaded to hand over to the woman's husband. Too often the husband is himself unwilling and embarrassed by all these female 'goings on'. This is where the fathers' class or couples' evening classes in which husbands meet each other in a group is of great benefit, as once the husband can feel that this is the manly thing to do and that other men do it, he may begin to offer more positive support to his wife.

I am often asked if I believe in insisting on husbands helping their

* Melanie Klein, *Love, Hate and Reparation* (London, Hogarth, 1953).

wives. This would be unreasonable and an unjustifiable intrusion on the marriage. But everything should be done to make the idea of helping her as attractive as possible. This includes an easy, relaxed atmosphere on the subject and praise and encouragement.

Fear of pregnancy, dread of labour, whether it be of sheer pain, laceration, of giving way and losing control, or of being subjected to humiliation, ridicule or exposure, generalized tension, worry about the baby, hatred of herself or of the child *are all problems for the marriage too*, and they can only be solved within the context of the marriage. A great deal is to be gained by a man and woman undertaking preparation together, not only in the woman's ability to adapt herself to the stresses of labour, feeling she has rehearsed it all well beforehand with his support, nor only in the help he can offer at the time, but for their closer understanding of each other.

Pregnancy is—or can be—an occasion of spectacular emotional growth, involving as it often does a series of crises as the expectant mother gradually comes to terms with her new identity. The emotional vulnerability and instability of the expectant mother are often observed facts in our society. It is, as it were, a second adolescence. Anything we can do to make this transition easier will be for the good.

On this front, within the context of a woman's whole psychosexual life, advances in the field of prenatal education must now come. So far from confining itself to teaching a set of physiological tricks, preparation for childbirth can teach a woman how to trust herself—a trust that should go far beyond the mechanisms of labour alone, and should involve not only education for the experience of birth but education of both parents for the demands of parenthood.

Underprivileged Women

8

Underprivileged Women in Childbirth

'It can't be done.'

'We haven't the space. . . .'

'These mothers wouldn't understand; they're uneducated—illiterate really. . . .'

'We just haven't got the staff to cope with these numbers. . . .'

'Not enough privacy. . . .'

'It's a very old hospital—built a hundred years ago—and it simply isn't suitable for us to be able to do this sort of work. . . .'

'They really . . . *enjoy* suffering. You'll never change them. That's the sort of culture they come from.'

Too often remarks like these stop us helping women prepare for childbirth and parenthood: women who have not had the advantages of education or money, but who have as much right to receive this teaching as any middle-class mother. Of course hospitals are ill-adapted to this form of counselling and group work, and we know that it will not be easy. But the challenge is there!

The challenge is not simply to instruct women in the anatomy and physiology of the reproductive organs and in techniques of adjustment to labour but to help them towards something which is even more valuable: discovering possibilities of choice, of voluntary decision and action, of self-direction, and of what those in the middle class think of as basic human dignity and responsibility.

Middle-class women are still striving to achieve a sense of personal responsibility and awareness in childbirth. But they have at least the opportunity to be articulate, to verbalize their feelings, and in many countries to 'shop around' until they find an obstetrician and a hospital who take their views into account.

The poor and uneducated cannot do this, and may not even be able to put into words what they want. If they criticize hospital procedures it is often simply in terms of not giving the comfort aids which they have learned to expect from their traditional untrained peasant midwives—the warm towels and anointing with oil, the fumigations and binders, the careful disposal of the afterbirth so that evil spirits cannot claim it, or the protection of the newborn from powers of darkness by clothing it in special colours or bathing it in special liquids. What they are really saying, perhaps, is that the experience of birth has not been integrated emotionally into their total life experience and the values which are meaningful for them; that they felt loneliness and isolation and the lack of warmth and understanding, and were deprived of the communication through touch which all people know who live in large families in crowded conditions, and those who say through physical contact those things which they cannot express in words.

The very poor, whether they are South American peasants or the urban poor of a great city like Chicago, often feel that events sweep over and through them like the wind and that they have no more control over them than over the climate. Trapped in an economic situation from which it appears that there is no escape, it seems to them that there is little or nothing they can do to change events or to placate the fates, the gods, or those others, *them*, who control their lives. They are as likely to have this attitude about birth, and the prevention of unwanted births, as about sickness, death and poverty itself. Moreover, for people who are economically and socially powerless, the ability to make a baby is the only power they know. This is why childbirth is an especially significant keypoint in the underprivileged woman's life.

Social revolutionaries try to motivate the underprivileged towards initiating change. But perhaps the real revolution has to start in a man's or a woman's attitude towards themselves, and themselves in relation to others, and begins with the ability to foresee, comprehend, plan and prepare, and then adapt his or her behaviour to changing circumstances. In this it is not only the economically impoverished who are deprived but also all those who because of skin colour or culture lack opportunities for social mobility and for getting an education to equip them to face the tasks which life presents.

Before starting to teach, instructors will obviously first obtain books which describe the culture from which the people they will be teaching come. Studies in sociology and anthropology, even novels, may provide this background.

It would be helpful to arrange to meet social workers, teachers and nurses who have done work with this cultural group and who can give more firsthand information. Endeavour first to meet some of the people you will be teaching in a small group in a private house or other relatively relaxed and informal atmosphere, so that you get to know some members in advance by name, and can also discuss with them what they expect of a course in preparation for childbirth and what they would like to learn. A health visitor may be able to arrange to take you on her rounds so that you can be introduced to some potential members in their own homes.

Amongst those who are living at or near survival level, and for whom having enough food on which to feed the children is the prime concern, it is to be expected that notions of motherhood will be largely confined to providing the basic necessities of life for the family. They cannot be bothered with subtleties of morality, and the functions of motherhood are all summed up in the ability to nourish. Among Jamaican peasant mothers and the urban poor I found that when I asked women What is a good mother? the answers provided by those who were really desperately poor were all given in terms of feeding. Only when the woman had a little more did she add 'and keep them nice', 'wash them clothes', 'keep them clean', and she needed still more before she could say 'make them grow up good' or 'teach them the Bible'.

For those of us who have enough to eat it is difficult to realize just how much the concept of motherhood has to be pared down to its basic essentials when one is living at hunger level. How much further removed still are all the concepts that have become associated with preparation for childbirth and the skill of a woman in: keeping control of the situation, being mistress of herself, understanding what is going on, handling contractions or training in neuro-muscular control! Such women are simply not interested in these ideas; they are utterly irrelevant to them. It is not so much that they cannot understand them as that they do not touch the realities of their lives and the struggle for survival.

When a woman has children who never quite have enough to eat at any meal of the day, who cry with hunger and beg her to give them food, or children who are forced to live in shack or slum conditions in which they are often not quite warm enough, who play at the side of a dangerous road, eat the paint from the crumbling walls, or are in danger of fire from poor electric wiring, or from the infectious delinquency of neighbourhood gangs, she has little interest in avoiding what she may see as more or less inevitable pain which she is required to tolerate for a few hours of labour. But probably every woman responds to any offer of help to enable her to become a better mother; she will understand very different things by this, but it is a promise that triggers off a positive response in her. Because however impoverished the conditions under which she lives she is concerned about her children and wants to be a good mother. Those involved in education for birth must remember this. Our task is only justified if we can go beyond the hours of labour and help women with their families. Part of this work concerns education in family relationships. But among the really impoverished much of it must be purely practical and provide assistance in referring to the agencies which can give aid, for ideally education for birth should find its place within a coordinated network of social services.

For many people who have little control over the forces of nature and who feel at the mercy of powers which are not susceptible to the technological manoeuvres at their disposal, magic and witch-craft help to give some semblance of control over those processes and incidents in life which involve most risk and danger. There is in magic a careful and internal logic which can be entirely consistent given the premises upon which the magical system of belief is based.★

★ See E. E. Evans-Pritchard, *Witchcraft, Magic and Sorcery among the Azande* (London, O.U.P., 1937).

One of the processes which involve most risk is that of *becoming*, of entering life, and it is not surprising that the transitions of pregnancy, birth and neonatal existence should often be hedged around with taboos and practices which are semimagical, and seek to protect the child during its difficult journey into life. Indeed in many societies in which the child is most at risk, the first days, weeks or months are spent in relative seclusion. It is in a transitional state of existence, and is not yet accepted as a social being; its life is too precarious to risk the suggestion that it is expected to live implicit in giving it a name. So there is usually an interval between birth and the rituals by which the mother, also in a dangerous state of existence, is cleansed and purified and birth and those in which the child is baptized, circumcised, or even dressed and taken out and submitted to the gaze of strangers.

In many societies the dangers which can befall the baby are attributed to the evil wishes or the loving possessiveness of ghosts or ancestor spirits, and the things which are done to protect the newborn are devised to afford a shield from this sort of activity from the other world. These important formulae for the baby's protection may consist of dressing the baby in certain colours, hanging charms around it, covering its head or mouth to prevent evil entering it or—as with Mexican babies—its spirit popping out between its lips, leaving beside it an open Bible—as in the West Indies—or a metal talisman, burning incense to attract good spirits, purging or bathing of the infant with special concoctions—as in many parts of South America—or cleansing or sweeping of the room in which the child lies. They may also involve treatment of the placenta and of the umbilical cord so that the child may prosper in its future life. Frequently, as in many parts of Africa, the placenta must be quickly and completely disposed of, so that no witch or other evil spirit may get possession of it, and hence of the child's spirit or fate; or, as in West Africa, it may be buried under a special tree which is henceforth the tree of the child's life. Similarly the child's nail parings and hair must be destroyed, often by fire, to avoid them coming into the possession of those who could do the child harm.

In modern hospitals mothers may be dissatisfied, but feel embarrassed at expressing their worries, because the child or its placenta or body products are not being safeguarded in these age-old ways, and yet the woman knows that such ideas are considered superstitious and outmoded and feels ashamed that she should have such thoughts.

In many modern hospitals women may have not only little encouragement or opportunity to express their fears but the very dehumanization of the whole conveyor-belt procedure—even when labour is easy—can itself reinforce *the sense of loss* which often comes with the birth of a baby, however much wanted and however loved. For the change of role from bride to mother, from being a girl to being a 'grown' woman, finally culminates dramatically in labour and delivery. A woman who placidly adapts to the changes of pregnancy may yet find the birth of the child, the resulting rapid changes in her body, and, above all, the fact that she now has to cope with a baby outside her that demands attention (and not one that could be automatically carried and nurtured within her own body) too great a challenge. Particularly is this so if the girl is still in reality primarily a daughter to her own mother, so that she cannot see herself in the image of a mother, and reacts to the child's crying as if she herself were the child demanding attention rather than being able to react as a mother and pick up, comfort and feed the child.

The birth of a baby, although it gives something to the mother, must also involve the loss of an old self. Different cultures and sub-groups within cultures, as well as different family norms, encourage varying modes of expression of these images of the self. Before we understand what motherhood means to a woman—not only what it gives her but what she loses—we cannot really comprehend either the problems that adjustment to parenthood may involve for her or what the child represents for her.

As the child grows older the way she holds it, the frequency and quantity of feeds, their abrupt or gentle termination, her manner of clothing and cradling the child, the way in which she attempts to discipline it or avoids formal discipline, and the phase of develop-ment at which these things are done, and at which she expects response are all patterned by the society of which she is a part, or in the case of the immigrant woman, of the two societies in which she stands, perhaps unsteadily—with a foot in each. The nucleus of this pattern consists in the social expectations of what a child *is*.

In those societies in which grandmothers frequently take over the care of children, or in which the grandmother is expected to give advice to and guide the young mother, it may be useless to teach the mother alone about modern baby care. If child rearing is seen as a family affair, one at any rate involving mothers and grandmothers, it may be necessary to teach whole families or to have classes in which mothers and grandmothers are invited to attend together. Within immigrant communities where joint households are common the most practical approach to this would be to teach female relatives as groups, whether or not they are pregnant or have young children. Education of immigrant families can intensify a gap between the generations which ultimately reflects upon the care a child receives and is associated with a struggle for possession of the child between the mother and her mother or mother-in-law. The older woman feels her values are discarded, and feels isolated and lonely at a time when her children have grown up and she is no longer needed as she once was. It is just the time when new understanding and cooperation could result from teaching in which modern methods were based on understanding of old values, the new allowed to grow out of the old, and its relevance to lasting values demonstrated.

We all have fantasies about the ways in which our bodies work, their boundaries, their inner geography, the parts which are associated, those which actually link up physically with other parts, and the size of the orifices. Sometimes this picture is relatively accurate, but perhaps most of the mental image we have concerning our bodies is constructed from vague feelings, states of fullness and emptiness, of strength and weakness, of heaviness and lightness, of heat and cold and of being 'open' and 'closed'. The image is constructed, in fact, of physical sensations, states of physical being.

Yet it oversimplifies matters if we think of these images simply as the by-product of a haphazard collection of stimuli. All nervous, stimuli, whether they provide messages from the outside world from the periphery of our body, or from internal parts of the body, are signals to the brain to act or respond in some way considered appropriate to the sensation, whether this is interpreted consciously and rationally, or whether it merely triggers off a response which is habitual, customary, or even simply conventional. That is, all stimuli are interpreted in terms of a total pattern of expectations, a picture which gives meaning, 'sense' and order to all sensations. The brain always organizes them, and this brain is part of a person—and the person is part of a society. Even the sensations we consider most intimately our own, our personal feelings which we share with no one else, are in a sense social experiences. We classify and code, translate and explain these stimuli in terms of an image that we have of the world and of society about us, and of a body image which changes as we grow and through different experiences of our lives, but which is our basic sense of what *we* are as distinct from anybody else, and provides the foundations of our sense of personal identity. Without it there could be no patterning of social relations, no association or avoidance between bodies that are not *me* and the body which is mine, no relationships of closeness between bodies within the family, between mother and child or husband and wife, and no interaction rituals by which public order is preserved.[*] The body image is like an atom of each system of social organization, and it is to be expected that different types of social organization and different types of body image are likely to be linked together.

Thus the body image is not just personal and private. Especially is this so when we look at concepts of health and sickness and of cleanliness and pollution. These, in turn, are linked with religious or mythical explanations of why such things are, and sometimes even with whole heroic sagas of conflicts between gods and demons in which different parts of the body form the setting for the enacting of the struggle between the forces of good and evil.[†]

When a woman is in labour one is observing her in relation not only to the biological body that one sees there on the bed but with a fantasy body—her body as she knows it and about which she has hopes, fears, worries, unvoiced doubts, apprehensions and expectations. Her ability to accept what is happening to her physiologically, and to cooperate with the process, has a good deal to do with what

[*] See Erving Goffman, *Interaction Ritual* (New York, Anchor, 1967) and *The Presentation of Self in Everyday Life* (New York, Anchor, 1959).

[†] Claude Lévi-Strauss, *Anthropologie Structurale* (Paris, Gallimard, 1958) and Mary Douglas, *Purity and Danger* (London, Penguin, 1970).

she thinks is happening, with her ideas concerning her internal functioning and inner geography, and her feelings of rightness or of disruption and danger in reaction to the stimuli which are crowding in upon her from her own viscera and from her physical and social surroundings.

We know that this is so with the educated middle-class woman who has an approximately accurate idea of what to expect in childbirth, but who is uncertain of the exact meaning of the signals which she is receiving from the uterus, or from the pressure of the baby's head as it descends through the arc of the birth canal and presses first against the base of the spine, then against the rectum and anus, and finally distends and bulges through the perineum. It is not only the stimuli which are coming from inside her which can be confusing but all those other stimuli which are received from her environment and which are the direct result of the sort of care she is receiving and the atmosphere of the labour room. Taken all together, they can result in such a confusing kaleidoscope of sensations that the woman can lose her bearings, and, further assisted in this process by sedative and analgesic drugs given without tender loving care or without informed support and guidance which can help her to control the situation, she can become disoriented and give way to panic and a crisis of anxiety.

The problems can be even greater for a woman whose body image is in conflict with body functions and treatment required by the hospital staff, and who comes into an environment for which she is ill-prepared, and where she is uprooted from all that is familiar or comforting in her own home environment.

The expressions which one sometimes sees on the faces of women in a maternity ward—noncomprehension, fright, and even unquestioning resignation, as if they are caught up in a process of which they can have no possible understanding—may reflect the tendency in some hospitals to concentrate solely on the contracting uterus and set aside the needs of the woman of whom it is a part. But for all the emphasis on technical matters such as monitoring uterine activity and fetal heart rate, if the woman's emotions are neglected or ignored, her anxiety can alter, and even completely inhibit, uterine function. Many of the emotions which can affect a woman in labour are related to the body fantasies concerning the whole process of pregnancy, childbirth and delivery.

Fundamental to each individual's body image are concepts about cleanliness and defilement and those parts of the body which are considered 'dirty' and to be kept hidden, or which are for general social presentation. For Western society as a whole, and in Mediterranean cultures, the upper part of the body is considered relatively clean and the lower part relatively dirty (whereas for Indians one side of the body is clean and the other side dirty). To expose the lower part has traditionally been considered shameful, especially for women.

Women often find it difficult to talk about their ideas about their bodies with doctors, even when they get the opportunity, and may even feel that it is improper to do so. In many ways a doctor may collude with women in setting the scene by which, through draping and isolating the lower half of the body from the upper half, and often through the use of evasive terms such as 'your waterworks', 'your tail', these parts of the woman's body become the doctor's property, not hers.

Researchers and health educators working with those of lower socioeconomic groups often feel that they are sailing close to the wind when they talk about gynaecological and obstetric subjects, and find that they have to find a way round a barrier of prudery. In England, one group found that not only did some respondents express astonishment and annoyance at being asked to talk about their insides but some indignantly made comment such as: 'If I had been interested in my body I would have gone in for nursing or St. John's [first aid]'. It was the doctor's business to talk about the uterus and vagina, and nothing to do with them.* In fact to get too involved and to focus attention on the part of the body which is appropriately called by some women *my privates* is verbally to expose that which is hidden and to reveal that which should be secret *from the woman herself.*

Where women customarily breastfeed without self-consciousness

---

* W. O. Goldthorp, W. Hallam and J. Richman, 'Medical Knowledge in Gynaecological Patients—A Study of the Patient's Understanding of her Illness and Treatment', *Br. J. of Sexual Medicine* (1975).

or deliberation, exposure of the breasts for this purpose, if necessary in public, is rarely considered shameful. In other societies, naked breasts are considered provocative, and women may find it difficult to think of their exposure for the purpose of feeding an infant as anything other than embarrassing, and even dirty. Throughout the Moslem world, exposure of the genitals to a male doctor, however well qualified and however necessary his function, may always involve a residue of shame, and in many hospitals women doctors have to be available to examine women patients.

Ideas about bodily secretions vary between cultures too, and this also relates to ease of lactation. When the dominant motif in the culture is to deodorize, purify and replace with perfume all physical secretions, whether their source is the armpits, the mouth or the vagina, as it would appear to be throughout most of the United States,* this tends to be accompanied by predictable attitudes to the inhibition of lactation and to attitudes towards engorgement which involve taking the baby off the breast as soon as there is any discomfort or difficulty.

In other societies the dominant motif may be the duality of *hot* and *cold*—the dangers both of fever and of a drop in temperature, which themselves are derived from the medieval European concept of humours. This can be traced back through Galen to Turkish and Egyptian sources, a concept which spread with the doctors who travelled throughout Europe from the Middle East. The effective treatment of any physical or mental ailment may then be defined in terms of raising or lowering of the temperature of the blood, and only those practices which seem to do this, as in drinking hot or cold potions or having hot or cold packs, may seem at all relevant to the patient's condition. Closely related to this are beliefs concerning hot, spicy foods and mild, bland ones—the hot foods being considered suitable only when there is some coldness in the blood, and the mild foods suitable when there is heat in the blood.

Puerto Ricans living in New York believe that health consists in achieving a balance between bipolar categories of hot and cold and dry and wet, and during the postpartum period women do not eat

* Vaginal douches on the United States market include some labelled 'champagne' and others scented with verbena or raspberries.

cold food since the uterus is considered to be cold at that time. So all food and medicine must be hot.*

In still other societies, beliefs concerning *stopping up* and *unstopping* may form the main pattern for the control of health and sickness. In Jamaica I observed a general theme in which health consisted of letting the body's substances flow, of somehow keeping them moving and of ensuring that all the ducts and passages were not blocked, and in which illness meant that secretions were stopped up or the interconnecting internal tubes were plugged by growths or by poison of some kind. The art of the healer and to a large extent that of the Obeah man, or witchdoctor, was to discover the source of this blockage and, by the administration of herbal medications, by massage, fomentation and fumigation, to clean it out. Because Jamaica is a very complicated society in which ideas from all the countries who traded and owned slaves overlie traditions brought but very dimly remembered from the coast of West Africa, these theories exist side by side with others concerning heat and cold and with the blood being too *rich* or too *weak* which seem to owe their origin to medical books brought over by the eighteenth-century plantation owners and used for medical treatment of their slaves.

Interspersed and overlapping with these main theories of disease are others again, probably having their source in Africa, in which illness is due to the evil wishes of another, and the action of ghosts, or *duppies*—who must be placated, charmed away, or somehow overpowered by magic, amulets, charms, incantations and ritual designed to ward off evil. So the West Indian has a rich tradition, stemming from different cultures, concerning medicine, and the West Indian woman in childbirth may have very precise ideas about what ought to be done and what avoided, ideas which, although they may not accord with those of modern obstetrics, are yet sufficiently varied to form a basis for further explanation from doctors and nurses, and all of which can without too much difficulty be linked up with present-day methods, if only they have some knowledge of the labouring woman's body image and will give the time to help her understand.

* A. Howard, 'The Hot-Cold Theory of Disease', *J. of Am. Med. Ass.*, Vol 216 (1971).

Ideas of this kind do not simply concern notions about ill health; they also define and form a framework within which normal physiological function is perceived. In fact one can ask What happens when you breathe? or Where does your food go after you have taken it in through your mouth? What happens to it? The answers, or pictures drawn, indicate again these fundamental motifs. Often people cannot find the words to describe these functions, and if we are to gain understanding of how these processes are perceived we must use an oblique approach in which, little by little, we piece together the various aspects of the body image like a very complicated jigsaw. Nor is it a single jigsaw, for the images of children and adults often differ greatly, and those held by men and women are always different, if only because they have different subjective experiences of their bodies because of their difference in sex.

The investigator working in a birth control clinic can obtain a good deal of material on women's body images if she will take the time and will encourage women to express their doubts and worries. I found that simply having a wide range of contraceptive devices available, letting the women handle them, and asking them of each How do you think it works? and Would you like to use that? and using these as general leads for further discussion taught me most about women's ideas concerning those parts of their bodies which they cannot see, and the whole inner geography of the abdominal and pelvic regions.

Similarly the attendant observing a woman in labour can use the opportunity not only to soothe or guide but also sometimes to ask Where is the pain or tightness or ache? or whatever it is the woman is finding it difficult to cope with, for example, What do you feel there? What is it like? and What is happening, do you think? This is where the investigator who is not in the position of the all-knowledgeable doctor or nurse can be at a distinct advantage, because if she fills the role of a companion in labour rather than as a healer or teacher, her questions and requests for information can arise quite naturally, do not seem out of place, and are not based on the assumed premise that everything the patient believes is likely to be erroneous, and that it is she, rather than the woman on the bed, who should be giving information. There is thus a strong argument for using labour companions who are not in uniform, and manifestly not part of the hospital hierarchy, to obtain this sort of material, and the sociologist or psychologist who has herself borne children can form a useful part of the labour team.

In many societies women fear that the baby can rise up out of the abdomen into the chest. This in some ways reflects concepts of the uterus being able to work clear of its moorings or be shaken loose into the body cavity, and with the theories of hysteria associated with this. Many things may be done to 'keep the baby down'. In Japan women used to tie their sashes extra tightly beneath their breasts. In Latin America women may bind their breasts firmly with tight shawls or strips of fabric during pregnancy for the same reason. West Indian women may tie a string under the breasts or, if they are too modern for this, may do up their bras extra tight.

Middle-class women from these different cultures will be more like middle-class women anywhere than like the peasant women and the urban poor who live in the same country, and these beliefs survive merely as old wives' tales which they smile over.

But one must not underestimate the force of old wives' tales, for however much they may be cause for amusement in daylight, they can be renewed with something of their old power in the hours of darkness. The pregnant woman unable to sleep or wakened from sleep by heartburn, the kicking of the baby inside her or by her own disturbing dreams, is particularly vulnerable to these half-dead ideas about what happens when the expectant mother raises her hands above her head or is frightened by a mouse. Discussion can be initiated best not by asking What do *you* believe? or What do *you* think? but What have you heard can harm the baby during pregnancy? and Are there any other things you have heard people say about what is good or bad for the baby while you are pregnant? Is there anything you can remember people saying about things that are good and bad for a woman when she is pregnant, not doctors or nurses, but ordinary people—older women for instance?

In labour itself not all women are convinced that the baby is going to emerge through the vagina. Most of us have heard tales of girls who thought the baby would be born through the umbilicus.

More common still is the conviction, reinforced by sensations of pressure against the rectum, that the baby is coming out of the 'wrong' hole or that the mother is not having a baby but wants to empty the bowels.

Commonly experienced sensations may be interpreted by the labouring woman in terms of the body image in which the baby can come up into the chest. When a Pakistani woman vomits, a frequent experience in the late first stage, and which she is very likely to do if she has eaten the special sweetmeats which are prepared to give strength to the labouring woman, she may interpret this as an indication that the baby has 'come up'. This is for her a signal for the husband's female relatives, who are the usual attendants of labour in the villages, to lean on the fundus to 'keep the baby down'. When she is in a modern hospital, or has emigrated to a country where she has none of her husband's female relatives to assist her, she may overreact to vomiting because she then feels stranded without suitable help to keep the baby in its right place and may appeal to nurses or doctor to press on the fundus in the same way. For the Jamaican woman the signal is a different one. She is likely to panic at the first signs of the expulsive reflex, which comes initially as a catch in the throat. She tends to interpret this sensation in the throat, as her breath is held involuntarily, as an indication that the baby has come loose and that a hand or foot is sticking in her gullet. Given the body image which she holds relating to childbirth and the sensations she experiences, this is a perfectly logical deduction.

Many customs which involve the use of tight binders or shawls over the top of the abdomen, and the Latin American and rural North American manoeuvre by which two women stand one each side of the labouring woman pulling alternately on a strip of cloth tied over the fundus in order to move the baby into the right position for delivery, can be related to this body image in which the baby can come up rather than down.

Thus the many fragments of belief about childbirth which exist only as old wives' tales now, once formed, or in some societies still form, part of a total body image. We can understand their significance only if we treat them with some respect and try patiently to unearth and piece them together with as much precision as if they were precious fragments of archeological pottery. Because they are intangible ideas, products of the human mind rather than material artefacts, they are no less worthy of gentle handling and careful reconstruction.

9

A Teaching Course with the Needs of Underprivileged Women in Mind: A Possible Approach

The following are intended as themes to explore, not sessions in a class syllabus. They are not meant as a blueprint for teaching in general, but as one person's approach to some of the problems presenting themselves with those expectant mothers who are not particularly interested in education for birth, but who attend an antenatal clinic, perhaps waiting for some time before they are seen by doctors, and with whom preparation could be done.

I am not sure that it would be good to provide a really exhaustive guide for teachers, even if it were possible. As the reader will be aware from reading Chapter 3, I believe that the essentials of what we are teaching are conveyed more in the manner of our teaching, in the atmosphere we create in the class, and in our caring and understanding than in the communication of a massive quantity of information and techniques. So teachers should not feel that they have to get in every detail of the suggestions which follow.

There is a good deal to be said for not thinking in terms of classes at all at first, but for going round talking to each woman individually, or to small groups, and making personal, friendly contact. This procedure has been found successful in some hospitals in the United States, where, for example, nurses working with Spanish-American, Black and Indian mothers in Texas find that in spite of being told that these mothers do not want antenatal classes, and that it will be impossible to interest them, motivation is not lacking when women are approached, one by one, about classes. In one Boston hospital an enthusiastic doctor found an empty cupboard off the main clinic waiting area, and sat in there with plenty of visual material, seeing two or three women at a time. Frequently the problem of getting a response from mothers of lower socioeconomic groups seems one of such magnitude that antenatal teachers find that it is more than they can begin to tackle alone, and need to look around for other helpers who can form part of a team. Some public health nurses in the United States are using student nurses as resource partners and potential educators, since many of them have a special concern for low-income patients. Other teachers find that when working with adolescent mothers there is an advantage in having assistants of the same age, and once series of classes are moving former students can be used in this way. Elsewhere women of the Black Panthers started courses for other women in the movement, which were advertised by a display in the store front of the Panther Headquarters, with a large and beautiful photograph of a Black couple giving birth to their baby together, and the question 'Do you want a birth like this?'

The first thing is to get attention and do something so that women sit up and take notice. One has to break through tremendous lethargy which settles over an antenatal clinic where women have to wait for prolonged periods. Interest might well be caught with the use of a doll and baby box, described on pages 69–73, preferably with a doll of the same physical type or colour as most of the women in the clinic. An audience will quickly form round a Punch and Judy show or puppets of any kind, and the antenatal teacher who is to attract an audience in this situation needs to have some qualities of showmanship. Or, it might be possible to have someone demonstrating techniques of handling labour in the middle of the clinic. Throw down a mat and pillows and show what it is like for a woman who is trying to escape from each contraction as it comes. Then, 'Now this woman knows what she can do to help herself!' and act the part of a woman responding to contractions with relaxation and breathing. One starts in at any point at which curiosity can be aroused, and proceeds from there. As an antenatal teacher working under conditions such as these you might carry small teaching aids with you all the time in the clinic so that you are ready to stimulate interest and to demonstrate at any moment. You may look silly, and feel very self-conscious about it at first, but the larger purpose for which you are working is more important than your personal comfort, and you will soon be able to carry it off with poise and a smile!

Note that alternative expressions, depending on culture group of participants, are shown thus: ....../....... These are by no means complete, however, and many other images will suggest themselves to the teacher.

How the Baby Started

Using the *Birth Atlas** emphasize sizes and relative sizes. The teacher might say: 'The woman's egg is not really like the egg you have in the kitchen. It is smaller than the head of this pin. It is called the ovum.' 'Enough male seeds could be put in this tin (a kitchen cake tin or small wastepaper basket) to make all the babies in the world today.' Other vivid material of this kind is obtainable from *The Everyday Miracle*† and *The First Nine Months of Life*,‡ and can be used both about fertilization and fetal development. Describe shape and size of womb/uterus; show an avocado pear or fig, stalk end down; place it in correct position on your own body. Either decide to use the term *womb* throughout teaching or clearly explain that *womb* and *uterus* mean the same thing. Women can get the idea that two organs exist side by side. Since women are likely to hear the term *uterus* used at least in labour, it may be wise to introduce them to the term in classes.

Then the unselfconscious demonstrator can turn into the uterus, and *acts ovulation* (see page 75).

Discuss *conception*, and provide some sort of visual description of

* Dickinson-Belskie, New York Maternity Center Association.

† Lennart Nillson, Axel Ingelman-Sundberg, Claes Wirsen (London, Penguin, 1967).

‡ Geraldine Lux Flanagan (London, Heinemann, 1963).

it. One way of doing this is by demonstrating the lashing movement of the tail of the sperm with a rapid movement of the hand and wrist. Say that when seen through a microscope sperms look very much like tiny tadpoles. Then with arms in a circle raised above the head, demonstrate the shape of the mother's ripe ovum. With the right hand repeat the swift movement of the tiny sperm towards the ovum, and with a large movement of both arms open up the circle to embrace the sperm. 'And it joins with the seed'— and draw in the arms in a firm circle with a quick tightening action.

'Now new cells grow fast and the egg and seed which have joined together is going to grow into a baby. But it doesn't look like a baby yet. Through a microscope it looks more like a mulberry/ blackberry/raspberry (whatever is most familiar to women in the group). And all the time it is bouncing along the tube towards the womb, a bit like this: It takes about one week for its journey to the womb.' Move a ping-pong ball slowly along the arm from wrist to shoulder, with undulating movement of arm. Then move it across on to chest. Pause a moment.

'Now it sinks into the soft lining of the womb and it starts to grow little roots into the lining.' With the free hand slowly stretch the fingers to resemble roots. 'The lining is for the roots of this baby that is just starting to grow a bit like earth/dirt for the roots of a plant. The roots draw food from the womb's lining, to make the baby grow.'

How the Baby Grows

Large simple drawings of the fetus at various stages can be useful. Demonstrate the bag of waters with a doll inside a polythene bag, but emphasize that these are much larger than life-size. At three weeks the baby that is to be is only about the size of a small grape (and show grape, hazelnut or something similar), at four weeks the shape and size of broad bean/kidney bean with budding legs and arms, at eight weeks the size of a medium hen's egg. 'And at that time the heart, which will work for a lifetime, has begun to beat, and hands and feet are growing.' Discuss the function of the waters against shock; 'lapped in warm water'; even temperature. <u>Explain placenta</u>: 'The placenta works like a strainer/sieve'—and elaborate this theme as useful. Discuss drugs, and smoking. 'The baby does not like smoking and it is not good for it. When you smoke you force your baby to take in the chemicals from the cigarettes. Although baby does not breathe inside it is already practising making breathing movements and it has been discovered that when the mother smokes the baby's smooth, easy breathing-like movements are changed and get jerking and gasping.' Take doll out of bag and show it to mothers, complete with cord and sponge placenta, and let them handle it as they discuss. Use *New York Maternity Center Schuchardt Charts*,* backed with cardboard and preferably covered in polythene, held against your own body to demonstrate the relations of different maternal organs to the fetus and the changing dimensions of uterus. Discuss discomforts of pregnancy in relation to these changes, and what can be done about them.

Say what the baby can do at each stage of growth, and which parts are developed, for example sucking thumb, hiccuping, eyelashes, nails. Discuss the movements of the baby and *knots* (usually accumulations of Wharton's jelly) in cord, especially with West Indian women, who may believe that number of knots in the cord indicates how many children they still have to bear. 'The cord is like slippery, wet spaghetti. It would be difficult to tie tight knots in spaghetti, wouldn't it?' Discussion of fears about the baby, effect of maternal emotions or experiences on the baby, pregnancy taboos and superstitions can grow out of this. 'Has anyone told you that you should not stretch your arms over your head when you are pregnant? What do you think of that?', and the like. Describe *vernix* (like face cream or cottage cheese); quickening—'It feels like butterflies inside, and perhaps a bit like goldfish swimming round—some women think it a soft thudding or a little like a slight electric shock.' What do *they* feel? Discuss the baby's sucking and swallowing movements, too.

Explain how *twins* develop, especially important with mothers descended from West African peoples, as a large proportion of twins are born to these women.

* Obtainable from the New York Maternity Center.

Looking after Ourselves and the Baby Through Pregnancy

Talk about *diet* in early pregnancy as well as later on 'to make a healthy baby'. Relate this to phases of development and baby's needs for protein, iodine, iron, vitamins, and the like. 'What foods do you think are good?' Discover and discuss food prohibitions within that culture with sympathy *not* condemnation. Discuss alternative foods if these taboos are strong. Where culturally approved foods are believed to assist towards easy labour (for example fig juice in Latin America, almond oil amongst Moslem women, okra in the West Indies), accept without criticism. The psychological benefits of taking these foods may be great.

Discuss *hormonal* ('"special juices" in the blood') changes and other physiological adjustments in the mother and 'the work of change' that this means for her body. 'Do you feel any different in pregnancy?' Discuss rest and fatigue, encouraging the women to talk together to work out how they can get some rest; changes in breasts and the ducts—'passages like many little rivers full of milk'. Describe the nipples—'holes like the spray of a watering can nozzle'—and the benefits of breastfeeding. Discuss the comfortable positions in intercourse. (It is important to know some common terms used by the people being taught. West Indian women, for example, may refer to intercourse as 'having my exercise' and to orgasm as 'feeling sweet' or 'having a discharge'.)

Discuss social services available to help low-income families and others.

Our Bones and the Way We Stand, Walk and Sit

Introduce the pelvis as 'the bony cradle within which the baby grows'. Let them track their own pelvises and discover capacity for movement of different kinds, after you first have demonstrated on yourself. Make sure they can all feel them and can rock and tilt the pelvis. Talk about height of the fundus, and engagement—'lightening', as 'the baby going down with its head like an egg in an eggcup'. Discuss posture in relation to the position of the pelvis.

Cradle rock and *cradle tilt.* Practise gentle and rhythmic *exercises for pelvic mobility*, without elaborate gymnastic preparations, but quite simply, sitting on firm chairs. The counter-pressure of the chair helps the women to get the feeling of 'tucking the tail under' when pelvic rocking. Pelvic tilting can be performed with alternate extension and bending at the knee of each leg. Resistance to exercises is often met on the part of Asian women, particularly when it involves pronounced physical movement. Exercises on a chair, at least at first, are less threatening.

Wings touching. Practise exploring all possibilities of movement in the *shoulders* and follow this with shoulder circling, and pressing the shoulder blades towards each other 'like angels' wings', and then releasing them.

Try *belly dancing*, or the Hawaiian 'trip around the island', preferably with slow, languorous music, but music appropriate to the culture group. Stress smoothness and gentleness. Some mothers may be able to teach the teacher.

All exercises should have easily remembered names and women may themselves suggest suitable ones.

Prenatal Care

What happens when you go to the clinic? Discuss what the doctor and nurse do to help during pregnancy, and why—abdominal palpation, blood pressure, checking urine, blood tests, chest radiograph, vaginal examination, sonar scan. Explain how to 'breathe out and go soft' for examinations, and practise this. Define unfamiliar terms, for example *lochia*.

Labour

Information about labour and what it feels like *precedes* any instruction about breathing and relaxation.

Discuss the signs that indicate that labour is going to start soon—heaviness, 'like a coconut between the legs', ache in thighs, low backache, increased vaginal discharge, perhaps slightly bloody, the 'show'. Explain frequent Braxton Hicks contractions and how they occur throughout pregnancy and are felt usually after about the seventh month. Describe *nesting* activity; they will probably all have stories about friends who have experienced this.

'But the only sure sign is regular tightenings of your womb, increasing in strength, lasting longer and longer, with the space between getting shorter and shorter. After this has been happening for an hour you can believe that you really are in labour.' 'Also the waters may leak or pop.' Explain that she should tell doctor if this is so and go to the hospital, because the 'cork' has come out of the 'bottle' and she is ready to start, whether or not the womb has started doing its work yet. Discuss when it is a good idea to go to the hospital in terms of their individual circumstances and different kinds of labour.

What Happens when Labour Starts and How Does the Baby Get Out?

Demonstrate the knitted uterus with the flexed doll inside. Explain *dilatation*. Demonstrate the shortening of muscle fibres rhythmically with a movement of hands, fingers extended and pointed downward, then slowly and regularly flexing progressively as if drawing the cervix up and open. Then take the doll out of the knitted uterus and put a balloon inside and inflate it. Place a ball, an apple or orange in front near the 'cervix' and demonstrate dilatation of the cervix. Discuss what contractions feel like and use *multiparae* for comments if possible. Show the doll against your own body and in the plastic articulated pelvis to demonstrate usual positions of the head. Can they feel with their hands any parts of their babies' feet, buttocks, back, head? Help them get to know their own babies in utero.

Use your fist in a sweater sleeve to indicate how the baby's head is pressed through the cervix—'as if you were pushing your head through a rather tight polo neck sweater'.

At this point emphasize rhythmic patterns of all harmonious physiological activity—the heart beating, breathing, defecation, *and* labour. Talk about 'letting the womb do its work' and the value of relaxation.

Teach simple *relaxation*. Show contraction and release of your own biceps. 'What happens to the muscle when I tighten it?' Get them to feel their own. With women in pairs, show them how to test each other, so that they get the feeling of alternately released and contracted muscles not only in themselves but in another's body. With Indian women, concerned about immodesty, or others who are shy, again it is less threatening at least to start relaxation practice sitting on chairs.

Use suggestion and scenes of tranquillity to which they are likely themselves to be accustomed. If you cannot think of any appropriate ones, let *them* make suggestions. 'When do you feel most rested and peaceful?'

Proceed from this to studying *parts of body most difficult to relax* and use imagery to increase neuromuscular awareness and ability to release tension—a hairdryer on the scalp to achieve relaxation of muscles of the head, heavy pendant earrings for relaxation of the jaw, smelling a sweet scent (get suggestions; it could be fish and chips, rosewater, incense, or anything that gets the desired result) for relaxation of the central muscles of the face, heavy gold rings on fingers for relaxation of the hands, wearing a new lipstick for relaxation of the mouth. Note that in this one is building up not only skills in relaxation but pleasurable awareness of different parts of the body.

Practise different *positions for relaxation*, and relate these to possible use in the first stage of labour, for example sitting on a straight-back chair, sitting in an easy chair, leaning against a wall, or standing with the support of another person or a table or chair, kneeling, squatting, on all fours, propped up on a bed, dorsal lying (not a good one), side lying, lying in a front lateral position. Discuss and practise possible comfort from gentle and slight pelvic rocking in suitable positions.

How Muscles Work

Refer back to what happened when biceps were contracted: 'The womb is a bag of muscle, the biggest muscle in your whole body. It is bigger than any muscle in a man's body. Bigger even than the muscles of a champion boxer. It will go on working beautifully when all the other muscles are relaxed. It contracts without you having to work to make it tighten.' Discuss the value of relaxing all other muscles to let the uterus work uninterrupted.

With mothers well propped up, lying on their backs, so you can see their faces, and they yours, with plenty of cushions in back, including the small of the back and behind the neck: Practise *alternate extension and release* of muscles of hand and feet. 'Your brain is telling your body what to do, rather like sending a telephone message down to the muscles, but even quicker.'

You might then go on to practise contraction and release of different parts of the body on a signal from members of the group, who take it in turns to instruct. 'You notice how you can control your bodies and get them to tighten and go soft very smoothly and easily now. You have to learn how to do it. Most of us can work with our bodies best in labour by first of all learning how to tell different parts of our bodies to go soft.' In this way women are introduced to the art of *differential relaxation*.

You may wish to proceed from this to the differential relaxation and contraction of limbs, separately and in combination, letting a partner check that there is complete release, for example, of the arm when the other arm is contracted, released, contracted and released. This can turn into *the game of not letting your right arm know what the left one is doing*. The woman who is assisting closes her eyes, and at a secret signal such as the teacher raising and lowering her hand, the women practising neuromuscular control contract, and then release, then contract again. Does the partner know when the other arm is contracted? The same can be done with the legs.

With such activity, which involves laughter and a good deal of movement, earnest concentration is best followed by a period of quiet resting and residual relaxation 'listening to the sound of your own breathing. Next time we shall talk more about breathing, because it is with your breathing that you can help your baby to be born'.

How To Breathe in Labour

Even though other subjects may run over, and these headings are not intended as separate lessons, here the teacher would be wise to allow a space and to start a fresh lesson on the subject of breathing.

Discuss breathing in terms of waves or mountains, with spaces or valleys between, depending on geography familiar to members of group. 'Slow breathing over all the little waves/easy hills is good.'

You demonstrate this. Then practise *slow costal breathing*, letting them work in pairs, feeling each other's lower ribs swing out, shoulders relaxed. See that they do not gulp in air nor tighten the shoulders. 'Breathe out! Concentrate on the breath *out*, and let the breath in look after itself.'

Discuss how difficult it is to breathe easily if the chest wall and shoulders are tight. Demonstrate poor breathing, with raised shoulders, emphasizing discomfort. 'Here is a woman all dressed up for a party with a new dress on that's much too tight', and act the part. Do *shoulder release exercise*, circling backwards, and then alternately shrug shoulders 'see if you can touch your ears with your shoulders' and release.

Follow this with a *chest release exercise*. 'Imagine you have on a bra which is three sizes too small' (or another garment familiar to members of group). Describe its appearance, shape and texture—bright pink, with rubber, large hooks and eyes, does up at back. Act the movements with them. Encourage them to get the last hook done up. Then 'All right it's off. Relax!' Get them to observe a good feeling of relaxation. Then do slow breathing exercises again.

Demonstrate and practise *light* (upper costal) *breathing*, using the finger tips resting lightly on the upper chest, and feeling slight movement in the upper chest wall, or with the partner's hands resting on the upper back. They can do this with each other and by themselves.

Move up gradually from slow breathing to shallow chest breathing, keeping the respiratory pattern smooth, partner's hand moving from outside the lower ribs up slowly to the sternum or upper back and then down again.

Then they do the same without help from their partners, your hand regulating the rhythm and depth of breathing. Remind them about the relaxation they have learned, and let them discuss whether they are well relaxed when doing it.

Teach the *leg-squeezing technique* to simulate uterine contractions. This is best called by some term such as *labour rehearsal*. The woman relaxes in a comfortable position and the partner gradually contracts her fingers over the upper leg as if this were a labour contraction. It should not be done on a leg in which there is a varicose vein. In that case select an arm instead. The instructor starts with easy, half-minute contractions, and the subject 'breathes over' them. At the end of each contraction she is asked to give a long blow out, a 'resting breath'. As women become adept at this instructors increase both the length and intensity of contractions. In later rehearsals they also practise making contractions with two peaks, others which seem to be fading away, but then return, and still others which start and then stop. Point out that in early labour contractions are often very smooth and regular, but in the late stage of 'opening up' they can be like steep cliffs or walls. This is the single, most important exercise to prepare for labour, and one which I always suggest is practised by husband and wife together. Repeat this practice at each subsequent class.

Talk about and demonstrate *overbreathing* in late first stage. If women are panting heavily ask them to visualize a leaf moving up and down very lightly or even a piece of tissue paper or a balloon. Describe sensations of hyperventilation—pricking in hands and feet, giddiness, even blackout, hands going tight with cramp, and what to do about it if it occurs. (Breathing out into cupped hands so that one inhales again some of the exhaled breath, or breathing out into a paper bag and breathing in exhaled air from it.) Explain that with overbreathing some chemicals important in the bloodstream are being flushed out by the panting, and one needs to 'go soft' and breathe more lightly.

What Labour Feels Like

'How do you think you will feel when labour starts?' Talk about feelings in the late first stage of labour, using experiences of the multigravidae. Recapitulate what happens during the first stage, using the *Birth Atlas*, and then show what happens during the second stage. The illustrations are best painted in primary colours for clarity —all maternal bone red, muscle green, placenta blue, and the like. Discuss in particular the sense of confusion, frustration and defeat which may threaten the mother in *transition* between first and second stage. Pushing too soon will not get the baby born more quickly, but will waste energy. Demonstrate with a doll, lie, attitude, flexion and extension of limbs, presentation, finishing by reenacting correct and most usual positions of baby. Techniques for putting over material of this kind are discussed on pages 70–3.

Talk about posture for the second stage, a rounded back position with the pelvis at its widest, head forward, shoulders relaxed, and why it is necessary. Demonstrate this and let the pupils practise.

Demonstrate *breathing for the second stage*. Sometimes they have seen mammals giving birth. Discuss what they have seen. How did the dog, cat, sheep or other breathe? Get them to practise holding the breath comfortably for twenty seconds (*not* pushing for twenty seconds), and check each person once in her bearing down movement, with one's own hand against lower abdomen, which should bulge forward and down if she bears down with a piston like movement from above downward 'like firmly and smoothly pressing toothpaste out of a tube' or 'stiff egg white through a pastry bag' or some other suitable image . . . 'letting the movement pass right through your belly into the vagina, till you feel yourself opening up below'.

Talk about the feelings of the second stage and delivery and about excitement. Demonstrate the curve of the birth canal and different sensations which occur as a result of pressure of the baby's head against different parts of this canal, demonstrating this visually with hand movement. Baby's head is 'like a large orange' pressing down. The vagina is opening up 'like a concertina'; it can get much larger. Then warmth, tingling and stretching around the vagina. They can get this feeling of stretching by opening their mouths and pressing with a finger on either side of the lips. Practise pelvic-floor release while doing this. 'Open the door for your baby to be born'. '*Give* birth to your baby.' Think 'I am giving life to my baby.'

Act the part of a woman who is not coping well in the second stage—strained throat, chin flung up, shoulders tense, buttocks tightened, legs contracted. Ask the class members to tell you what is wrong and to help you get it right.

Working through Transition

Transition is a bridge between the time when the womb is opening and the time when we can push (methods of teaching about transition are discussed on pages 226–30).

The theme is transition as a sign of *progress*. The most difficult time of labour, when things are not going to get worse and worse and worse. Describe feelings, exasperation, despair, exhaustion, fear of pain, backache, thigh ache, the tight band of contractions pressing in all round the abdomen and small of the back, drowsiness, disorientation. Emphasize the problem of apparent timelessness, unfamiliar surroundings, strange people.

Stress that classes teach women to understand what is happening, and what the staff is doing to help and, most important, how the woman in labour can help herself. She 'isn't just lying there like a fish on a slab or jelly on a plate. She's *busy*'. 'The things we learn in classes make a sort of map, a map of where you are coming from and where you are going. There are signposts along the road so you know how things are progressing. One of the most important is transition.' Discuss legs shivering, difficulty in relaxing, feeling cold, hiccuping, ache in legs, pain around pubis, very low backache, feeling rooted to the spot, nausea, possible vomiting, malar flush, tendency to breathe rapidly and heavily—watch for overbreathing.

Practise *blowing out* crisply and swiftly as if through straw or puffing a balloon away to cope with the powerful contractions and urge to bear down or both before full dilatation.

Practise the technique of shallow, light '*mouth centred*' *breathing* for the tops of difficult contractions, mouths open, lips soft, jaws relaxed, cheeks plumped up as if smiling slightly ('it can help a lot to smile, so practise smiling'). Check relaxation. If one loses rhythm or feels that breath is getting 'caught', blow out as previously practised.

Describe '*back labour*'. Imagine contractions with a repeated urge to push. Discuss the probable intense backache, long first stage, long transition and emphasize patience. Rehearse the technique of *mouth centred breathing interspersed by any regular rhythm of light blowing*—puff, puff, puff, puff, *blow*, puff, puff, puff, puff, *blow*. Demonstrate overbreathing. Ask the class members to help you get the breathing right. What can they suggest? Discuss this and then again the correct way of breathing so that this is the last thing left in their minds at end of class.

'Do you think it is worrying to go into hospital? What do you find worries you most?' Discuss what is done to help the mother and baby in labour, and how to work *with* those who are helping. Ask for experiences of friends, neighbours, relatives who have had babies. Discuss these fully as well as hospital procedures, and problems in communicating and understanding. Make sure that admission routines are clearly understood. Arrange a tour of labour and delivery rooms, if possible, and meetings with other members of staff.

Find out if anyone wants her *husband* or partner to be with her in labour. 'Are you planning to have anyone with you to help you in labour?' If the prospective fathers are not already participating ask 'Would you like them to learn how to help you? What do you think your husband could do to help?' Discuss this. Can a special meeting be arranged at which those men who were not able to be in classes can be taught simple techniques of support? Although many men in Western and other cultures resist becoming involved, once they see that there is a positive role for them they often take on responsibility gladly. A Los Angeles childbirth educator said that although they anticipated difficulty with Spanish-American husbands, 'we are tremendously oriented to husband-support techniques and this seems to appeal to the Latin man's strong sense of masculinity (*macho*)'.

Labour Rehearsal

Emphasize that each labour is different, and one cannot know exactly what will happen. Labour is always an adventure. This is when other women's labour reports may come in useful. Have a few newly delivered mothers tell about their labours, what helped, how they coped.

Families (*including Looking after the New Baby*)

If there are other children in a family have a discussion on their feelings about the coming baby—how to let them feel bumps and kicks. Discuss jealousy, how natural it is, and how to help the displaced baby. Talk about the husband's attitude to the baby.

'What do you think he feels about it?' Is it all pleasure? Is there something else? Get them to talk.

Demonstrate a baby bath and changing of nappies with a *real* baby. Talk about hygiene and cleanliness, getting ideas from group. Discuss postnatal care of the baby—care of cord stump, and the like.

Have a nursing mother and baby in class to discuss the advantages and how she has dealt with problems, and to nurse there if practicable. Describe the let-down reflex, the feelings a mother may have when the baby is at the breast. Talk about the appearance of a new baby, with photographs of a newborn, and about initial reflexes— 'What is a good mother like?' Investigate how to work out household routines suitable to different kinds of families. Discuss the basic needs of the newborn, and emphasize that they are different from those of an older baby, a toddler and an older child. Discuss physical loving and tenderness, security, comfort, reassurance, but also freedom to explore, stimulation. Include where to find expert help with family problems, and have addresses ready. (You must know cultural backgrounds and most common problems and child-rearing customs to make this discussion really worthwhile.) With an introduction *beforehand*, show a film of birth and have a discussion afterwards.

Continuing personal contact is necessary for classes which cover this kind of material to be really effective. One nurse working at an adolescent prenatal clinic gives each mother her home phone number and invites her to contact her any time with questions. In this particular clinic staff meet with the prenatal teacher after sessions to discuss how they can better help specific mothers with severe problems. Team-work in this way is important. At another clinic catering for adolescent expectant mothers, a lunchtime conference session for nurses and prenatal teachers is held every two weeks to learn about all new mothers coming through the clinic and to discuss ways in which they can more effectively meet the needs of those with particular psychological, social or high-risk obstetric problems. One teacher telephones all women ahead of time, and lets each know that she is at the clinic to talk about the birth with them, and to show exercises which can make them more comfortable in pregnancy and breathing techniques which will help in labour. She mentions the names of other young mothers coming to the sessions if they are from the same school or neighbourhood, makes an appointment for a time together, always adds that she is looking forward to meeting her, and when the girl arrives she goes out to the waiting room to welcome her.

The Skills We Teach

10

In Progress

Twenty years ago antenatal teaching was very much a matter of exercises, whether they were mainly relaxation or breathing exercises or ones designed to improve body mechanics in pregnancy and the postpartum period. Some of these exercises were thought at the time to make labour much easier.

The first that were introduced were those of Dr Kathleen Vaughan, based on her obstetric work in India, where she had observed that women often had their babies very easily, even though many of the mothers were malnourished, and attributed this to the squatting postures customarily adopted. Minnie Randall, and after her, Helen Heardman, invented and developed the new skills of obstetric physiotherapy, the latter incorporating the teaching of Dick-Read into her method and teaching slow deep breathing, moving the abdominal wall out and in with inhalation and exhalation, and relaxation in the front lateral position.

Psychoprophylaxis introduced still more exercises, based on the Pavlovian discovery of conditioning and deconditioning in experimental animals, called relaxation by a new name—*decontraction*—and invented new types of breathing rates and levels for different phases of labour. Under the impact of psychoprophylaxis breathing exercises proliferated, so that wherever antenatal classes were taught there seemed to be some new variation or complication of exercises, and as I travelled on lecture tours across the United States, and in Canada and the United Kingdom, I was often asked if I myself taught. 'Huff and puff', 'Slump and blow', 'Choo-choo breathing', 'The sigh', 'Levels A, B, C and D', 'H out, H out, Hoo-hoo', 'Sss-sss', 'Tune-tapping' or whatever. I do not know if the mothers were as confused as I was. Certainly it all tended to be very noisy, and labour wards hummed with activity as women busily breathed their way through contractions, often to the consternation and dismay of midwives, who sometimes saw these exercises as rites which were exhausting for mothers and midwives alike.

Disassociation was the main theme for all these exercises, with the idea that a woman could concentrate on some activity so hard that she was distracted from pain. Undoubtedly this worked for many. Women were taught how to block pain sensations, but along with them they tended to cut themselves off from many other sensations, including sometimes help and instructions coming from their obstetric attendants, and also, because of the rigid conditioning and exercise drills, the inner rhythm of uterine contractions which I believe should always guide the labouring woman's responses, whether these involve her breathing rate and levels, or pushing, or anything else that she is taught to do in childbirth. Some doctors called this 'brain-washing', and perhaps it was. Such brain-washing may be justified if it gets a woman through a labour with confidence when otherwise she might be unable to cope.

Now there is an opportunity to move on from this sort of exercise, and many teachers have done so, if only because as the whole idea of childbirth education has been accepted as valid, not only in the community, where it started, but in maternity hospitals, increasingly women are encouraged to use the skills they have learned in classes and to handle their contractions in whatever way they have learned. There still exist hospitals where women who have attended classes are greeted sardonically with 'Oh, you're one of *them* . . .', cruelly with 'You think relaxation will help. You just wait! You'll be screaming your head off before you get much farther!' or, with grim satisfaction, 'I've never seen it work for anyone *yet!*' But more and more midwives and obstetricians expect their patients to be doing *something* positive, and not just lying there hoping it will be over soon. So the content of our teaching has become more important than the fact that we are allowed to teach anything at all. It would be a pity if, as hospitals become more tolerant of antenatal teaching, we did not take the chance to adapt and modify and to make of childbirth education something more sophisticated than the early gymnastic drills provided.

Many experienced antenatal teachers have moved away from the old muscle-'stretching' exercises that were first invented for use with the original English psychoprophylaxis. (Who wants to *stretch* their muscles, anyway?) A good many have also turned away from the Dick-Read/Heardman type of squatting, because this often impedes the circulation of the legs in late pregnancy. It never achieved any widening of the pelvic outlet, as was first thought, unless it was a habitual posture adopted from childhood, as it is amongst many African and Indian women. We have also come to distrust the exercises, ostensibly for the strengthening of the pelvic-floor musculature, which involve contraction and release primarily of the adductors and glutei, and even of the calves of the legs. They used to be introduced with the instruction to 'cross your ankles and press your knees together'. Doing exercises like these, even though superbly well, can mask the woman's inability to hold on to a real pelvic-floor contraction.

Other athletic exercises involving a high degree of muscular effort, which may exhaust the pregnant woman, have also gone the same way. No longer do we believe that energetic and exaggerated arching and humping of the back in an all-fours position is good. Excessive strain can be put on the sacrolumbar ligaments in a minority of cases where these are already stretched by the advancing pregnancy.

What are we left with? And where are we going from here? Is there any room for exercises in childbirth preparation? And if so what are these? What is the range and purpose of the exercises we use? For me these fall into six categories: those for relaxation, breathing, focused concentration, the second stage, good posture and body mechanics, and genital and pelvic-floor awareness.

Teaching Relaxation

Progressive relaxation should include exercises in both differential and residual relaxation. *Differential relaxation* is release of some parts of the body whilst holding other muscles contracted. *Residual relaxation* is complete relaxation, letting the whole body go limp and loose. The distinction between these two types needs to be made, and a link made between such exercises and real-life situations, so that each pupil becomes more aware of the tensions to which she is subject in her daily life and her *spontaneous reactions to stress*. To limit the exercises taught to purely mechanical drills which entail an exercise session of a few minutes each day and then have no connection with anything else the woman does, or the sort of person she is, is to restrict the effects of our work unnecessarily.

The first kind we might examine are those based on acting techniques invented by Constantin Stanislavsky (the Russian theatrical director who created what has become known as the Method school of acting). My Stanislavsky-based exercises, involving the use of the imagination, aim to make a bridge between the class and the real-life situation.* In exercises of this kind the pupils act situations involving muscle contractions; and they should be of such a kind that many of them can be practised by the husbands too:

A. simple tasks, based, for example, on domestic and office activities.

* Some of these are described for the use of expectant parents in my *The Experience of Childbirth*, revised ed (London, Pelican, 1974).

B. tasks involving some emotional stress.

C. finally situations involving great stress, both general ones which can be shared, and other purely personal and private ones, which may be the subject of recurrent fears or dreams—things which the woman herself knows worry her. These may or may not be communicated to other members of the class and to the teacher, depending on the woman's own wishes.

With this approach to relaxation the woman begins to understand what happens to her body when she reacts to stress with tension. She learns that she can control, disperse, and finally let this tension slip away by concentrated and active relaxation. This sort of teaching of relaxation is useful for stress situations in everyday life, for household and family emergencies, as well as for labour.

When first practising these exercises it is a good idea to get members of the group really to act and move. Later on they learn that static muscle contractions can reenact these events in the same way without involving movement. It is these static muscle contractions which encase us within our bodies—some, of course, more than others—and which form each individual's own 'body armour'. Hence anxiety or apprehension, or a tense striving to succeed, can create involuntary contractions even though no movement is made, no action performed.

Exercises of types A, B and C are:

A.   1 squeezing stiff egg white through a syringe to make meringues
     2 carrying a heavy tray
     3 ironing
     4 putting on a bra two sizes too small
     5 struggling into jeans two sizes too small
B.   1 driving, about to overtake—a car coming in the opposite direction sweeps round the corner at speed
     2 making a cake in the kitchen; your mother-in-law comes in and asks if she can help
     3 you are buttering toast and suddenly see that the milk is about to boil over
C.   1 lying in bed at night you feel very unhappy about

something and are trying not to cry, and trying not to let your husband see you are crying

2 waiting at the station booking office for your ticket, the train is just about to leave; it is desperately important that you catch it. The doors are being closed, people are saying goodbye, and the clerk *still* hasn't given you the ticket.

3 recreate in the imagination an actual situation which has caused you great distress personally.

Each exercise should be followed by complete relaxation and a few minutes peace before embarking on the next. It is important to do this so that residual tension is not carried over from one exercise to the next.

Touch Relaxation

In Mrs. Hope's class none of the mothers quite understand the breathing and relaxation exercises, and only two of the meetings are given over to them. We lay on tidy pallets struggling with our tensions, and many were confused. No one was touched at a point of tension. Again, I felt the purpose was undermined by an excess of gentility and deference. Doctors don't care to touch patients at a point of tension either, I have noticed, although they will acknowledge its profound effect upon our physiology. Perhaps it is too deep for them. It is often a local source of diffuse pain, the knotted muscle, but don't touch it! Attack the headache indirectly with the prescription pad. And this tactile aversion is sometimes carried to such an extreme that the result is rather like setting a broken arm with the injection of a wonder drug.*

People respond in different ways to being taught relaxation, and a method that works well with one may be useless with another. Approaches to teaching relaxation ought to be as varied as the woman to whom we try to teach it. In my own teaching of relaxation I have found it useful to attempt to adapt my teaching to what appears to be the needs of each particular woman. If we think only of the verbal imagery appropriate to the teaching of relaxation, it is clear that any image may fail dismally for a woman with whom, because of her

* Charlotte Painter, *Who Made the Lamb: the Intimate Journal of a Woman's Pregnancy and Childbirth* (New York, Signet, 1966).

personal experience and memories, the words conjure up a situation which is unknown or preposterous or uncomfortable. I remember suggesting that complete release of muscles of the scalp felt as if one's head was warm—as if one had just come out from under the hair dryer, and a student flinched at the thought, and protested, 'But I can't *bear* that! I *hate* that feeling!' The teacher therefore needs to be aware of the response in each particular instance, and at the same time develop, with the help of the students, new images and a store of relevant similes.

We need not depend upon verbal stimuli alone. Our culture is, or has been up till now, a highly verbal one, and we tend to teach through and with words when sometimes there are other means of communication open to us. We need not leave these other ways of making contact only to chance or spontaneous impulse—such as when we smile or lean forward, or reach out a hand.* Nonverbal methods of communication, which are taking place all the time alongside the purely verbal language, and which may intrude on and actually alter the message of verbal communication, can be examined and understood so that we can use them deliberately, with forethought and skill.

In experimenting with using nonverbal means of communication as a systemized method of instruction in neuromuscular release, I have found this simplest to base on the spontaneous way in which husband and wife touch each other, because they like to, and because it gives them pleasure, comfort, reassurance, erotic delight and companionship. I have an abhorrence of the sort of antenatal exercise which entails leaping around doing a parade-ground drill for B-Day. Although some women find it very cheering I cannot see how, apart from pepping up the circulation, it can have any possible effect on a woman's effective adaptive responses during labour.

Labour is not the be-all and end-all of life, and to practise only with the few hours of labour in mind is to limit our teaching of relaxation unnecessarily. After the birth, what then? The woman is holding a baby in her arms. How does she hold it? When she is

* See for example Michael Argyle, *The Psychology of Interpersonal Behaviour* (London, Penguin, 1967).

feeding the baby, changing it and bathing it, and when she holds her toddler, greets her mother-in-law, copes in the kitchen or does her housework, writes her thesis, or deals with illness in the family, when she is driving a car, shopping or offering help to someone in distress or dealing with all the maddening, chaotic, nerve-racking, ear-splitting crises in a family—How is she then? Relaxation should be tackled at the level of ordinary, everyday living and be something women can incorporate into life, rather than merely an exercise.

A woman has to begin with space in the twenty-four hours when there is time to concentrate on achieving release. The obvious place is before going to sleep at night, and the best place is bed. Yet on the whole antenatal teachers have been a bit suspicious of exercises in bed and have thought they could not be done properly there. But it is the time and place where husbands and wives normally meet, however separate their paths during the rush of the day, and therefore when the husband can quite naturally be involved in helping.

Think of what happens as the husband or wife says What sort of day has it been, darling? and reaches out to touch the other. They may not even need the words—in a happy marriage the couple has their own private language, consisting of phrases, odd words, terms of endearment, ways of touching, or back-rubbing, sitting in firelight, or listening to music—in which they are able to relax. In a marriage where they have not achieved this, or where they have forgotten it, perhaps pregnancy is a time when they can learn, or relearn, the art.

Touch Relaxation is not just a matter of whether she can relax her right arm. It is concerned with both physical relaxation and also relaxation of the mind. It was one of my own students, who had been in and out of mental hospitals, who brought this home to me most vividly: she was an enthusiastic and hard-working pupil, but I felt we had to go beyond sheer mechanical exercises and somehow fit the relaxation into her life and help her to make it a quite natural response to stress. After she had had her baby she wrote: 'You gave me the most precious thing of all, peace of mind.' It seems a tall order; but I doubt whether I should have been able to teach her anything at all, except a series of 'circus tricks' for labour, unless I had somehow managed to help open the door for her to find that for herself.

The basic grammar of this nonverbal language of touch is simple: Release *towards* the touching hand. This is what you do spontaneously when someone you love touches you. At the same time it is important that the husband learns that he should touch with a relaxed hand, slowly, moulding his hand to the shape of the limb or any other part of the body on which they are working (occasionally he finds it very difficult to learn this). Thus it is seen as a *mutual* exercise in release, and there is never a question of the wife becoming a criticized pupil, subordinate to the husband; instead they are participating together in what is really not so much an exercise as a 'sensitivity response'.

She contracts a set of muscles, and when she is ready (not before) he rests his hand on the contracted muscles. The second he does so, she releases towards his hand. There are various ways in which this can be done, and it is a good idea to concentrate on parts of the body which the woman finds it rather more difficult to relax. The woman lies on her back, propped up and well supported with pillows in a warm bed, with support all up her spine, including the small of her back and back of her neck, and under her knees. She breathes out and relaxes completely. One system of exploring ease of release over different parts of the body is as follows:

1. She frowns. He slowly strokes her brow with the pads of his fingers from over the bridge of the nose out towards the temples. She relaxes.

2. She contracts muscles of the scalp and raises her eyebrows. He rests his hands on either side of the scalp. She relaxes.

3. She presses her shoulder blades back towards each other 'as if they were angel's wings and you could make them touch each other'. He rests his hands at the front of each shoulder. She relaxes.

4. She pulls in her abdominal wall towards her spine, at the same time tilting her pelvis forward. He rests his hands on the lower curve of her abdomen. She relaxes.

5. She presses her upper legs together 'as if you could hold a

sheet of paper between them'. He massages the outside of each thigh. She relaxes and her legs flop apart.

6. She presses her legs out, still flexed, but forcing her thighs apart. He massages the inside thighs, with a firm stroke down and a light stroke up. She relaxes.

7. She contracts the muscles of one arm like a wooden doll. He strokes slowly and firmly down her arm with both hands, one on the inside and the other on the outside. Her whole arm is relaxed.

8. Repeat with the other arm.

9. She contracts the muscles of one leg by pointing the toes up towards the ceiling and straightening the leg (this should not be done if it causes cramp). Slowly and deliberately, he moves his hands, one on either side of the leg, down the leg from the top to the ankle and holds her bare foot firmly round the instep. Her whole leg is released.

10. Repeat with the other leg.

The woman then turns on her side or in the front lateral, whichever is the most comfortable, and in this position:

11. She hollows the small of her back. He rests both hands firmly against either side of the sacrolumbar spine and she releases.

12. She presses her buttocks together 'as if you had a £5 note between your buttocks and someone was trying to take it away', and he rests a hand over the lower curve of each buttock, and she relaxes.

Each of these positions of tension can be related to specific common stress situations in which this tends to be the reaction, both in everyday life and in the different phases of labour, and to sensations of discomfort and to emotions. If they are not to be just exercises, it is vital that the teacher make this link. You can say, 'we often contract these muscles when . . .' *or* 'I notice I am inclined to tense up this set of muscles in a situation where I feel . . .', and the students can be encouraged to add to this from their own experiences. For example,

2 can be related to tension headaches

3 to build-up of tension in the late first stage of labour with resulting overbreathing and possible hyperventilation

5 and 6 to difficulty in relaxing in transition when there may be extreme coldness and shaking in the legs

7 to the best kind of help during difficult contractions in labour. Is it really very helpful to hold her hand? May she grip on it? What about stroking her arm, if she likes it to be touched (and some women hate it)?

11 to the sort of despairing bearing down when a woman feels she is not making headway, and contracts muscles in the back

12 to resistance to the odd sensations as the baby's head descends through the birth canal and presses against the rectum and anus, and then against the vagina. Both adductors and glutei may contract if the woman is resisting the sensation and finds it intolerable.

Touch Relaxation techniques also have an important place actually in labour and are a valuable means of the husband offering practical labour support, which does not involve nagging or even put the woman into the situation where she feels Who's having this baby— you or me?

The husband who is alert and sensitive to see the build-up of tension, however slight, can rest his hand on muscles involved, both between contractions, and, if the wife wishes it, at the onset of contractions. Here there must be ability to communicate easily, since touch can also be an intrusion and should only be used in labour when the woman finds it really helpful. Massage is a logical extension of Touch Relaxation.

It should be emphasized that once a woman has become skilful she not only can respond to the stimulus of her husband's touch with relaxation but can both use her *own* touch also to assist release and accept the touch of doctor and midwife as a signal for release too, although their touch is primarily exploratory and not aimed at providing the same stimulus. If a woman, previously tense, can discover the effect of releasing when the obstetrician examines her, and instead of 'drawing in her horns like a snail' can relax completely, the increased comfort she experiences and her doctor's surprise, provides its own impetus to perfecting relaxation for labour.

Experiments with a Relaxometer

The Relaxometer* is the simplest of a series of biofeedback machines, and can be useful in a private lesson but not in the class

* Manufactured by Aleph One Ltd, P.O. Box 72, Cambridge, England.

situation. In a class it acts as a distraction and pinpoints attention directly on one person who must feel that she is either successful or found wanting, depending on whether she can make the machine respond with a high-pitched whine or a low clicking, or even go silent.

One problem with using it is that the noise produced by the apparatus is in itself a cause of tension. For this reason the teacher should start it already at a steady clicking rate and a not unbearably high pitch. Some experimenting with the knob will help her to decide what seems to be a tolerable sound, and this is then what she should aim at in its subsequent use.

Because this is a machine we must not be misled in an admiration for technical apparatus into thinking that it is infallible. I doubt whether it actually measures relaxation in the sense of neuromuscular release and serenity of mind. What it does record is galvanic skin response and movement, however slight, in the limb to which it is fixed. It is possible to cheat it, however; I found that I could focus on an emotionally disturbing fantasy being careful to remain completely relaxed, and the machine could not detect the mental anguish. Similarly, second-stage type breathing of a very energetic kind does not necessarily raise the machine's pitch, and I found that I could bear down strongly and yet have little effect on the machine.

Nevertheless, I still think that for some couples the machine can be helpful in practising to maintain relaxation for labour, after an initial learning period during which the basic art of relaxation has been acquired. The following are two ways which I have used it in private consultation:

A couple came because the husband thought his second wife ought to learn something about her body before she had their son. It had to be a son. He was not interested in a daughter. She spoke little English and he took charge of the situation entirely, coaching her as if she were a rather dim-witted child, and giving us nonstop criticism of her performance. She was embarrassed, tense and frightened. 'She is my silly little girl, my baby. She understands nothing,' and a little later, 'my wife is neurotic, quite neurotic.' His wife smiled glassily and waited obediently to be taken in hand. I realized that I had to teach the husband before I could teach the wife, and that I had to teach him not what he thought he wanted to know—how to direct his wife's muscular control—but the very negative effect he was having on her and how he could replace it with more positive emotional support. The first step was to try to convey the pleasure and luxury of deep relaxation, and to give her constant praise to build up her self-confidence. When teaching couples Touch Relaxation it is obvious that men touch women in many different ways, depending on the nature of the relationship. In this case the husband thought himself rather an expert, but tended to attack her suddenly, with the result that she winced rather than relaxed. He wanted very much to be in the centre of the picture himself, so much so that he insisted that he lie back breathing heavily in an armchair while I rested my hands on his body and he showed me and his wife how good he was at it.

I produced the Relaxometer, deliberately set it very low so that the woman did not feel challenged, and simply talked her into relaxation. Gradually she relaxed more deeply and the machine went through the 'snoring lion' stage, and then fell silent. I told her gently that I would rest my hands on where the baby lay and where the contractions would pull and open the womb wide in labour. She would feel the light warmth and pressure of my hands and I wanted her to release *towards* the touch. We did this and the silence remained. I asked her husband to do the same, and immediately the machine started screaming. This was a hard lesson for him to learn, and I do not think he was under any misapprehension that she was responding with erotic excitement. She was reacting with apprehension and alarm to every touch of his.

It was only then that we could begin to discuss the special way of touching and of massaging that can assist relaxation, as distinct from all the other ways in which one can express oneself through touch, and he began to think there was something he wanted to learn too. We went on rehearsing very simple touch of this kind, first not using the machine, and then using the Relaxometer till he could communicate with her through touch without causing her anxiety.

I never had a labour report from this couple. I suppose they had a daughter. Whatever else I failed to teach them, I feel that the Relaxometer used in this way within the framework of counselling may have allowed them to make use of my teaching in the wider context of their relationship as a whole. It had allowed me to give the little jolt necessary for him to ask for help, not with what he thought he wanted at first, but with what was a basic difficulty in their relationship.

The other way in which I find the Relaxometer helpful is when a couple are practising simulated contractions together and he is squeezing a bit of flesh on her thigh. However expert the husband at checking her relaxation and working in detail over her body to test arms, legs, head and neck and elsewhere, it is practically impossible for him to do efficient testing when they are rehearsing labour contractions if at the same time he is acting the part of her uterus. With the Relaxometer he can concentrate on making the contraction and giving her verbal support, while the machine records any tensions building up during the contraction. It is important to begin with easy contractions and only slowly progress to ones which really involve discomfort. For the woman who is very apprehensive about 'going to pieces' with pain, it can be very encouraging to learn that she *can* remain relaxed while he is gripping hard. He for his part will almost certainly observe signs of tension, particularly in the face and neck, in muscles round the mouth and eyes, just before the rise in pitch of the machine. There is a time lag between the skin response and machine's recording, and he soon learns that he can actually predict when the machine is going to raise its pitch, just by looking at his wife. This observation of very early signs of tension is of great value for the support he can give her in labour, as then he feels confident in helping her even *before* there are any signs of tension obvious to an outsider.

12

Exercises for Increased Body Awareness

Many exercises for use in pregnancy are connected with the need for adjustment of *posture* with the increasing weight of the gravid uterus. Basic principles for good posture, whether in pregnancy or not, apply here. Exercises should aim at developing poise and a sense of well-being.★

I have found that there is a special advantage in developing a sense of *awareness of the pelvic region*, of the muscles around the birth canal and, associated with this, a feeling of physical rightness and harmony in this little-understood region of the female body. Exercises for the pelvic-floor muscles might be considered separately as being of overriding importance in childbirth education.

We are confronting age-old traditions of mystery and dark feminine secrets when we discuss with our pupils anything connected with their genital organs. In societies all over the world, menstruation, pregnancy, birth and the puerperium are linked with a mystique which is entirely irrational. In our own society it is often connected with dread of cancer. Blood flowing from the vagina, whether menstrual or puerperal, has often been thought to

★ Suitable exercises are described in Eileen Montgomery's *At Your Best for Birth and Later* (Bristol, John Wright, 1969), and in Margaret Williams's leaflet *Keeping Fit for Pregnancy and Labour* (London, National Childbirth Trust, 1969). Also available is a series of film loops by Margaret Williams showing breathing, relaxation, posture, lifting and postnatal exercises from Camera Talks, 31 North Row, London W1.

contain powerful substances which can endanger the lives of those coming near or touching it, or the woman from whom it is issuing, and to put her in a state of ritual danger. It is not surprising that women often seem to feel that they are under a primeval curse (witness the popular name for menstruation). This blood flow is also linked with ideas of pain, suffering and humiliation.

There is, therefore, room for exercises, always rhythmic and flowing, which increase in women a happy consciousness of this part of their body both as good, clean and right, and as under their control. This can have psychosexual effects much wider than those directly associated with childbearing, and these exercises naturally link up with those for teaching awareness of breathing.

Dancing involving full movement of the pelvic region, and alternating contraction and release of the glutei, abdominal musculature and adductors falls into this category. Girls familiar with modern pop dancing are at an advantage in this, and music can often be used to help. Belly dancing, if performed slowly and smoothly, is excellent. These exercises should also involve conscious contractions of the pelvic-floor musculature; they are so important that a whole chapter is devoted to them.

Often the pelvic-floor exercises are taught only in connection with defecation and emptying the bladder. Childbirth does indeed bring sensations closely connected with these processes, but to suggest that childbirth is simply a type of excretion and that the baby is a form of excrement is unfortunate. Many women feel disgust at the whole process because it seems so much like getting rid of waste matter. As a result they may expel the baby compulsively and without any delicacy or ability to 'listen to' their own uterine contractions in the second stage of labour; the main aim being to get it all over with as quickly as possible. There is here a connection to Freudian fantasies in early childhood in which the baby is conceived through being eaten, develops in the stomach and then is expelled through the anus. Such an image of childbirth, whilst natural to a small child, finds no part in the images of a mature woman who is receiving adequate preparation.

Childbearing is part of a woman's wider psychosexual life, and we can point out in passing that if she knows how to make love, she knows how to have a baby, but just as there are techniques in love-making, so there are techniques of adapting to labour, not all of them so very different from ones which may also be useful in intercourse. Some involve special sorts of movements and increased neuromuscular control of these areas.

Such exercises include gentle pelvic-rocking movements in different positions, so adjusting the degree of pelvic tilt, circular movements of the pelvis, both clockwise and counterclockwise; gluteal contraction and release; deep pelvic-floor contractions, including those supporting the uterus and bladder high inside and those around the base of the spine (ones which I usually sum up as 'kangaroo tail' exercises).

There is room for exercise sessions, and not only for verbal instruction and discussion in the class for preparation for childbirth and parenthood. But we should be sure in our minds of what we are doing with each exercise and avoid, above all, falling back upon rigid physical jerks or pursuing any course of exercises which does not directly help a woman to express herself more easily and rhythmically through the medium of her own body.

With this in mind we should be careful to avoid a drill-ground atmosphere when we introduce exercises and should concentrate on movements that we do *with* the group members. We might talk about exercises thus:

It is a good idea to do a few simple antenatal exercises each day during pregnancy since these encourage good posture and body mechanics, and can help us feel and look more attractive. A woman who carries herself well in pregnancy stands tall, with buttocks tucked in, weight distributed evenly over the soles of her feet, not on her heels, and the baby cradled in her bony pelvis rather like an egg in an eggcup [demonstrating this yourself].

There is no point in doing complicated exercises and no advantage in any that are very athletic. In fact exercises should always be done rhythmically, without straining, and without holding your breath. If they are so hard to do that you find yourself holding your breath it is a sign that they are too strenuous. It is much easier to get your figure back after childbirth, too, if you have kept in good condition and have not let your muscles sag by standing and sitting badly. It is also wise to avoid straight leg-lifting when lying on one's back, and any exercise which involves deep hollowing of the small of the back.

Brisk walking, swimming, dancing (but not in smoke-filled rooms), and any sport which you enjoy and do well, and hence with good physical co-ordination, can be helpful, provided you do not get exhausted. Balance and weight distribution change with advancing pregnancy and this may mean that certain actions you performed easily before become difficult and that you become clumsy. Although a doctor told me of a patient of his who was a tightrope walker in a circus till she was seven months' pregnant, I would not advise it, however frilly and all-disguising the skirt! Housework can be useful if you learn how to use your muscles effectively, without wasting energy or becoming tense, and if you do it cheerfully and with a swing. Polishing or scrubbing floors on all fours is especially good, since you get the weight of the baby off your spine for a while.

Some of the most useful exercises can be done while doing other things, and the most important of these are pelvic-floor muscle exercises which can be performed while standing at the sink, doing ironing, waiting to be served in a shop, or at a bus stop, or while sitting in a car at the lights, and every time you go up and down stairs.

Exercises which can be fitted into daily life without special sessions, or which are unobtrusive so that we can do them almost anywhere, are better than the kind we really feel we should put on a leotard for—and we are much more likely to do them regularly and often, anyway. The basic thing about exercises is that they should affect the way we *constantly* move—how we pick up the toddler or the vacuum cleaner, the way we make the bed or clean the bath, sit at a desk, or carry the shopping home—rather than being expected to do magic tricks for us. Getting to know your body in pregnancy, and leaning how to work with rather than against it, can also help towards quick and full rehabilitation after the baby is born, so that you hold yourself well and progressively improve muscle tone during the important six to eight weeks after the birth.

Exercises afterwards are not radically different from the ones for pregnancy, and many of the prenatal ones can be adapted. In hospital a physiotherapist will show you how to do the ones for the first postnatal days, and will give you a list of others you can add to them at home later. Do not try the whole list all at once, however eager you are to get your tummy flat and your waist back, since you can do more harm than good by not approaching them progressively. Aim at smooth coordination rather than physical jerks and, again, as in pregnancy, concentrate on the invisible pelvic-floor muscles, which are easy to forget.

The following are some exercises the antenatal teacher may find useful. Be careful always to explain *why* a certain exercise is done.

For Pregnancy

1. Blowing Out the Candle

(To keep tummy muscles firm.)

Lie on back, pillow under head, knees drawn up, feet apart and level with hip bones, soles of feet flat on floor near your bottom, hands resting on your abdomen. Breathe in slowly through nose, counting 1-2-3-4, allowing abdomen to expand. Then breathe out through mouth slowly, counting 1-2-3-4, feeling abdomen being drawn in as you do so, and when you feel almost empty, *blow* out remaining breath, as if blowing out a candle flame. (On counting 1-2-3-4, suck in abdomen firmly towards spine.) Hold it firm for a few seconds and then let your lungs fill up again.

Practise once a day when resting, six or seven times.

2. Belly Dancing

(For tummy muscles, general mobility, and as a treatment for constipation.)

Stand with feet a little apart, one foot slightly in front of the other. Rest one hand on your abdomen and one over your buttocks. Now move your hips round in a smooth rhythmic swing as if you were drawing circles or making a slow hula-hoop movement. Keep shoulders still. Notice how your abdominal muscles tighten and release as your buttock muscles tighten and release. Allow your knees to bend slightly. Then change direction.

Practise when dressing and undressing, for a few minutes at a time. This exercise can also be done to music. The timing should not be brisk, but rather luxuriously slow.

3. The Rag Doll

(For a straight back and toning of tummy and buttock muscles.)

Stand feet apart, about 20 cm (8 in) away from a wall, or it may be easier using a corner or door jamb. Drop forward like a rag doll, arms hanging, and the upper part of your body heavy. Your bottom should be just touching the wall. Adjust your position and start again if you are too far away or too near. Now gradually, vertebra by vertebra, uncurl against the wall so that one part of your back after the other is pressed back towards the wall. *Keep your shoulders relaxed* and don't 'pump' with them. Last of all your head comes up. Now you are standing straight. Notice the pull on your muscles.

Some women with little lordosis (curvature of the lower back) can stand absolutely straight against the wall. Others have a hollow back which cannot be entirely prevented.

Do this exercise once when dressing and undressing.

4. The Egg in the Eggcup

(To assist in good posture. This exercise can sometimes make a woman look two months' less pregnant than when she is standing lazily.)

Tuck in the buttocks, feeling as if you were curling an imaginary tail between your legs, and simultaneously lift the baby up with your buttocks and abdominal muscles as if lifting an egg into the eggcup of the pelvis.

To be practised at first looking sideways on in a full length mirror.

5. Wrist Push

(To tone muscles supporting breasts from above.)

Stand straight or kneel, legs apart, grip wrists with hands at shoulder level in front of you, elbows bent so that they form a rectangle. Firmly push skin of wrists up towards elbows, as if pushing tight bracelets up your arms, gripping as hard as you can while raising arms a little more with each push, till after five pushes your arms are just above your forehead. Then do the same thing with five pushes coming down to chest level again.

Repeat three times.

Exercises for Discomforts of Pregnancy

1. All Fours Exercise

(To relieve backache, get the weight of the baby off your spine and ease the strain on your back.)

Get down on all fours, with arms and thighs at right angles to your body as if you were playing bears, and do gentle pelvic rocking. Be careful not to let the small of your back cave in, as this sometimes increases the natural stretching of pelvic ligaments.

This exercise is a good one for advanced pregnancy.

2. Shoulder Rolling

(To relieve strain when there is upper backache in late pregnancy.)

Roll the right shoulder backwards and round in a smooth continuous movement, leaving the arm hanging loose and relaxed. Do the same with the left arm. Repeat with the right shoulder going forward, and then with the left going forward. Then work both shoulders at the same time, moving first one way and then the other for ten seconds each.

3. £5 Note Exercise

(For excessive elasticity of ligaments resulting in the tendency to stumble. This exercise will not make the ligaments any less stretched, but can help posture.)

Either lying, sitting or standing, and before getting up from a chair, sitting down or making any change of movement, press buttocks firmly together as if you had a £5 note between them and someone was trying to take it away. When practising, hold the contraction for ten seconds.

Another exercise to assist good posture in this case is number 4.

4. The Cat

(To encourage flexibility and suppleness if you feel heavy and stiff; and a useful exercise if you are tense and keyed up.)

Lying on your back in bed or on the floor, stretch as if you were a cat in front of the fire, wriggling and rubbing shoulders, pelvis, the length of your back, legs and arms against the bed or floor surface. Concentrate on getting your whole body moving slowly and sinuously. When stretching the feet, be careful to point toes up to avoid cramp. Then do a long breath out and relax completely. Lie quite still listening to the sound of your breathing for a few minutes.

Practise at beginning of rest period during day and when you go to bed at night.

[N.B.] If you find yourself wetting your pants when you laugh or sneeze, the *invisible lift* exercise (see page 178) will help.

If you are constipated, do the *belly dancing* exercise (page 169).

Postnatal Exercises

In the first week: Do exercise 1, *blowing out the candle,* as soon as possible after delivery.

Do the *invisible lift* exercise (see page 178), when feeling has returned to the perineum (if it was ever lost). Practise to the point of pain but not beyond. This will be a very slight movement at first if you have had stitches.

After stitches are out, practise interrupting a stream of urine. When you can do this effectively you know that your muscles are really strong again.

Do exercise 3, *belly dancing,* lying down in bed with your knees bent.

On the third day, add to these an exercise for the lateral abdominal muscles:

Leg Sliding

Lying flat on your back on a firm surface, draw one foot slowly up towards your buttocks, sliding along the bed or floor. Feel your abdominal muscles pulled in and your waist pressed down as you do so. Hold the position for a count of ten, and continue breathing. Then slowly push the foot back to its former position. Repeat with other leg. Be careful to keep the small of the back pressed flat against the surface.

Repeat five times.

On the fourth day, or as soon as comfortable, add another exercise for the abdominal muscles and waist:

Compass Swing

Lie flat on firm surface as in previous exercise, *waist pulled in towards floor,* arms bent and out at the sides. Pull in your abdominal muscles, raise your right leg and swing it over the left leg keeping it straight, till the foot touches well out at the side of the bed, and keeping your left hip and both shoulders on the surface. Raise your foot as high as you can in the air again, and swing back into its previous position. Repeat with left leg.

Repeat twenty times with a steady rhythm.

After this, do *housework exercises*:

Exercise 3, *belly dancing*, can be done when you are vacuum-cleaning and floor-sweeping.

Pelvic-floor lifting, can be done while walking up and down stairs, ironing, laying the table, and every time you change a nappy.

Exercise 1, *blowing out the candle*, can be done in a sitting or standing position, while mending, cleaning shoes, or watching television.

13

Teaching Awareness and Control
of the Pelvic Floor

There are two reasons why pelvic-floor exercises are important. Firstly, to increase neuromuscular control so that the musculature has good tone to support the contents of the pelvis during pregnancy and postnatally and, secondly, to increase the ability to open up and let go during labour so that minimal resistance is offered to the fetal head, and chances of needing an episiotomy or having a laceration are reduced.

Girls do not learn this sort of 'gym'. They shin up ropes and vault over horses in the gym and run with lacrosse and hockey sticks. Yet the very muscles on which general health depends are neglected: those vitally important in pregnancy, after a baby comes, during labour itself and for a woman's sexual adjustment.

A hundred years ago prolapse of the uterus and bladder were considerd an almost inevitable result of frequent childbearing. Women expected to have backache and a feeling that their insides were dropping out any time from the menopause on. And not a few younger women endured this also, especially after having a baby. The only cure seemed to be rest and a life of leisure; it was not understood that a muscle atrophies if it is not used. A newly delivered woman might expect her abdomen to be swathed in a binder and her legs to be tied together for a while in order to let the pelvic-floor musculature repair itself; or, if prolapse seemed unavoidable in middle age, a ring pessary was inserted to stop the uterus from dropping right down and protruding through the vagina.

Here are exercises or sensitivity responses which are suitable for all ages and conditions of women, whether they are eighteen or eighty. In fact with increasing age or with ill-health, and especially with the muscular inactivity associated with lying in bed, it is especially important to learn how to use these muscles and to maintain them in good tone.

Sometimes these same muscles go into involuntary spasm. This is typical of one situation of sexual misery called vaginism, when a woman contracts the muscles around the vagina during lovemaking, so making penetration impossible or very difficult and painful for both partners. Women sometimes suffer vaginism during a gynaecological examination, too.

Frequently it is not complete vaginism that is involved but an involuntary tightening which instantly contracts the ring of muscle surrounding the vagina. This may happen in any love relationship during the initial stages and is one of the clauses of secondary frigidity after childbirth (especially after an episiotomy). So for those suffering from involuntary contraction of the pelvic-floor muscles these exercises can also be helpful. It is not only learning how to contract but also how to release them that can be of value, and awareness and control allows both to occur at will.

The 'posture' of the pelvic floor is no less important after the child-bearing years are over. Slackness of these muscles and a feeling of one's inside dropping out, combined with low backache, are often associated with the tiredness and depression sometimes categorized by the term *menopausal distress*. It is not just a question of hot flushes —which are a matter of hormones—but of a mental attitude to parting with youth and oneself as potential bearer of a child. For many women depression is physically expressed not only in the sagging face and tense, hunched-up body protecting itself, but in sagging pelvic-floor musculature. For these muscles have an expression and respond to moods just as the muscles of the face respond spontaneously to emotional states.

So here is one of the most important parts of a woman's body. Because we stand erect and walk on two legs rather than on all fours a good deal of strain is put on the pelvic floor with advancing pregnancy, and the very fact that there are three openings in it, from the bowel, the urethra and the uterus further weakens the structure. Small boys love to experiment with controlling and cutting off the flow of urine, and are using their pelvic-floor muscles when they do. Small girls rarely seem to have any equivalent kind of game. But children are often aware that they can play with their pelvic-floor muscles in one way or another; as one child remarked 'Us can talk wiv our bottoms'.

So unaware are some adult women of their pelvic floors that we have to start by accepting that our pupils may know nothing about them at all. The woman experiencing difficulty in intercourse needs most of all help of this kind to be able to accept the genital area as a wholesome and acceptable part of her body. Teaching pelvic-floor exercises in the right sort of context is one way of doing this.

All sessions at pelvic-floor exercises, however brief, should finish with a tightening-up movement. We can point out that just as we do not go around with our jaws hanging slack or our eyes heavy lidded so we need not go around with our pelvic floors slack and distended. The important thing is to learn exactly what we are doing with them, in broad, sweeping movements, and also in much more subtle ways, so that we can respond appropriately in any situation. If intercourse happens ever to be uncomfortable we make it much worse by contracting the pelvic floor, for instance; the thing to do is to breathe out and relax and feel oneself go soft and welcoming.

Pelvic-floor exercises should not be taught as jerky winking movements. Ideally they should be taught progressively, just as we often aim to teach general relaxation progressively. Try to teach the ability to hold long, sustained, smooth contractions with poise and without breath-holding anxiety. I aim to teach gradual contraction, rhythmically and with control, and gradual release.

Beware of always teaching pelvic-floor exercises in terms of holding on to a bowel or bladder movement. We do not all perform the same sorts of actions when we do this, and if really under stress one tends to contract a great many more muscles than those necessarily involved. Moreover, as suggested in Chapter 19, it is unfortunate if we convey that our genital organs are primarily concerned with processes of evacuation, or that having a baby is just another form of pushing out waste matter.

Explain that the musculature is not much like a floor at all, but rather like a set of stage scenery, with the flats angled in different directions. If we think of the muscles in this way, rather than as a solid tray of muscle, the exercises become easier to do.

Exercises are best done every day, and if possible three or four times a day—I suggest as suitable times when one is washing up or going up or down stairs or standing at a bus stop. The exercise session could well be linked with a regular occurrence. After the baby comes, when the nappy is changed is a good time perhaps, or while feeding.

But in the last few weeks of pregnancy, and the first few weeks of the puerperium (although this very much depends on the degree of bruising caused by the delivery) or in cases of multiple pregnancy or hydramnios, the exercises should be performed lying down or, better still, lying on the back with the lower legs raised on the seat of an easy chair. This position takes the strain off the pelvic floor which has been subjected to stress.

To locate these muscles, imagine a pudding bowl slung from the pelvic girdle—a pudding bowl made of strong elastic and with three openings in it: the tubes leading from the bladder, uterus and bowel (the urethra, the vagina and the rectum respectively). The biggest sweep of muscles is roughly in the form of a figure eight round the vagina and the anus. At the point where the lines cross over there is the transverse perineal muscle, rather less important than the double circle of the levator muscle. Higher up inside are layers of pelvic floor muscle which support the uterus and bladder. If we are thinking about prolapse of the uterus or bladder the muscles on the outside are obviously the last line of defence, and we should aim rather at strengthening the muscles farther up inside so that women never get this 'dropping out' feeling, or the low backache and weariness associated with it. The whole muscle is an elevator, being capable of rising and of considerable range of movement, similar to the muscles around the mouth.

The Invisible Lift

I ask women to imagine that the pelvic floor is a lift in a large department store, and we are slowly going up four or five floors. By degrees all the muscles are pulled in, higher and higher up inside. It helps to empty the bladder first. We start off 'first floor . . . second floor . . . third floor . . . fourth floor . . . fifth floor . . . hold it. . . . Now see if you can get up one more floor. Good. Keep that for half a minute.' (The women who are doing this correctly are almost invariably either raising their eyebrows or tightening their mouths. It is only when a woman has become very skilled in differential relaxation, and does this deliberately, that pelvic-floor contractions are not echoed in the face.)

Then we let the lift go steadily down, floor after floor, till we reach the ground floor. 'Now we are going down to the basement, and I am going to ask you to let your pelvic floor bulge outward, as if you are helping your baby's head to bulge forward. This is what you will do during vaginal examinations in labour, and also in the very late first stage and the second stages of labour, to let the baby be born. And now we are going to finish the exercise by going up to the first floor again and leave it there with good pelvic-floor tone.' I suggest that they do this exercise regularly six or seven times a day, two or three times each session.

'Now let us concentrate sensation on the particular parts of the pelvic floor. The back one, forming the anal sphincter, is powerful and easy to move, although because all this muscle is interconnected, exercise of any part results in some movement of other parts too. This is normal. First, then, the muscles, the sphincter, around the anus. Hold on to it, and then relax. Now the vagina hasn't any sphincter like that, but there is a ring of muscle about halfway up inside which tightens the vagina and also draws it forward, tilting slightly upwards towards the pubis. Let us tighten that slowly and deliberately as if we were trying to hold a hazelnut inside. It is rather like a speeded-up nature film of flowers closing up into tight furled buds at night. Hold the contractions firmly.' Only when women have achieved this feeling can the teacher then add 'This is really what you do when you make a kiss inside when making love.' A few women are unaware of these possibilities until mentioned in the antenatal class; a remark of this kind will allow them to feel that they can discuss any difficulty of this nature, or anything else connected with sex, freely with the teacher. It is up to the teacher whether she feels she can handle this sort of material or not. For those interested and concerned this is the sort of remark that lets women feel able to talk about such things.

One can do all sorts of things with the pelvic floor. One can not only 'talk' but 'write' with it! I might suggest, 'Try writing Happy Birthday with these muscles. Remember to dot the i. As you move to the top of each letter your muscles are contracted; as you move down they are released. Remember to do generous loops and tails and rounded O shapes and you will get extensive movement.'

Then I point out that the highest level of muscles inside are at an oblique angle, just about under the hair line, and they can pull in these best by first of all tightening the ring of muscle, which in fact goes an almond shape as it tightens, and then pulling muscles up away from the hard lump of the pubis symphysis they can feel with their fingers. This is the muscle which is the first defence against pelvic-floor slackness. 'Rest your fingers on the pubic hair line and then pull in farther as if you can press the muscles up towards the bladder. You will feel another stratum of muscle contract, the layer which is important in preventing descent of the bladder. At the same time you will notice intra-abdominal pressure resulting from the tightening below.'

Exercises for muscles at the base of the spine 'where we would have a tail if we had one' I sum up as Kangaroo Tail Exercises. 'Imagine you have a great heavy kangaroo tail. Feel with your fingers the point at which it is attached, just between the buttocks at the bottom of your back. Now you are slowly, slowly going to lift this massive tail and hold it up, and then, just as slowly let it drop down on the earth, and if you are doing it properly and have your fingers in the right place you will be able to feel the muscles working.' Then I let any women who are finding this difficult feel *me* doing the exercise.

'Now we are going to swing this tail from side to side, and it will probably be easier if you move your jaws as well.'

It is important to exercise this muscle, not because it supports anything much, but because it can contract involuntarily in the expulsive stage of labour, or just before its onset as a result of uncomfortable pressure against the lower bowel. Some women panic at this point, and endeavour to hold in what they feel must be a very large bowel motion; they may worry about dirtying the bed or doing something disgusting. They often cannot believe it is a baby's head they feel. Or if they do, they are anxious that it must be coming 'out of the wrong hole'. Discuss all this and the emotional problems presented by these half-formed thoughts with women during pregnancy and show that release of these muscles, pressing down slightly towards the bed, will in fact help the baby to be born more easily and that holding back can only add to discomfort and even slow down the labour. Massage by the husband at this point with gentle pressure against this area may help the woman achieve release too.

Once women achieve skill at these exercises it can be pointed out that they are invisible ones, and that it is not necessary to contract the adductors or glutei to do them, as they will have learned from their own experience. 'Notice that you do not have to press knees or ankles together to do these exercises and that they need not involve any muscles in the legs or buttocks. Indeed, if you tighten up all over you can mask your inability to make the pelvic-floor muscles work hard. The important thing is to isolate them and work them alone.' Yet there is often an association between these groups of muscles and the muscle of the pelvic floor, and in labour it is also important to know how to release the adductors and the glutei.

To practise a gluteal squeeze preliminary to relaxation: 'Imagine you have a £5 note between your buttocks and someone is trying to take it away from you. . . . Now relax.' 'Now imagine you have a piece of writing paper between the tops of your legs and hold it in place by pressing your knees and legs together. . . .' Now relax.'

From there the teacher can do:

1. Gluteal contraction, held; add to it pelvic-floor contraction. Release pelvic floor. Release glutei.

2. Gluteal contraction; add to it pelvic-floor contraction. Release glutei. Release pelvic floor.

3. Contract adductors. Add to it pelvic-floor contraction. Release pelvic floor. Release adductors.

4. Contract adductors. Add to it pelvic-floor contraction. Release adductors. Release pelvic floor.

These may be very difficult to do at first!

All these exercises should encourage good circulation in the pelvic area and may, therefore, also be used in cases of premenstrual discomfort and heaviness.

14

Some Psychological and Cultural Aspects of Breathing in Labour

The way we breathe is closely connected with our emotions. Excitement, concentration, fear, apprehension, feelings of well-being or hatred, and sexual passion, all affect the rhythm and depth of our breathing.

The occasions on which we experience these emotions and the mode of their expression are in great measure created and dictated by society, which not only canalizes emotion, but actually initiates its expression within socially sanctioned institutions. The actors, however, are largely unconscious of the social origins of the emotions they feel, believing them to be personal and spontaneous. In many (but by no means all) societies childbirth is one of the important events concerning which, like the menarche, marriage or death, suitable emotions are socially binding on all concerned.

In labour the stimuli coming from the uterine contractions and from dilatation of the cervix act as signals to the brain—signals which are always interpreted by the labouring woman in terms of what she believes is happening in birth. These beliefs involve a map of the body world in which the individual operates, and of other people's body worlds, which is shared between women in any one society, is handed down from mother to daughter, and is social in origin.

Pain does not simply exist per se. It always means something to the person concerned and to the wider society of which that person is a part. It is related to past experiences and expectations, to the knowledge that fire burns, needles prick, knives cut, heavy weights crush, narrow passages split under pressure, and to socially recognized dangers implicit in the physiological processes of growth, injury and decay. In labour these signals can mean 'I am being torn apart . . . ripped in shreds; I am bursting; my back is splitting; I am being punished for sin; the baby is coming up into my chest to choke me; I am suffering the curse (or humiliation) of women; this shouldn't hurt, but it does, so something must be wrong . . . they are going to have to take it away'.

The dominant pattern of body images related to pregnancy and childbirth in any society will determine to a high degree just how these stimuli are organized by the brain and find their place within the individual's total body percept. Society, in the form of labour attendants—mothers and mothers-in-law, medicine men, witches, priests or obstetricians—reinforces these concepts at the time of stress by describing and interpreting what is happening in birth, myth, ritual (whether this is a peasant-type ritual or that ritual which can emanate from hospitals), chanting, dance and prayer.

So the stress of the repeated internal stimuli coming from uterine contractions may be accompanied and intensified by others coming from the environment. These may include different kinds of music, incantations, practices such as lighting a fire on a woman's abdomen or between her legs to smoke the baby out, or elaborate preparation for the relief of anticipated pain, physical restraint, solitary confinement, or baffling terms which suggest threat.

All over the world the late first stage of labour, when both the internal and external stressful factors are at their height, often heralds a period of overbreathing—in effect rapid, deep panting—which in some cases leads to maternal hyperventilation. In Germany, 75 per cent of a sample study of 141 women overbreathed.* In England, four groups of mothers—those who had not been in classes, and groups who had received training in psychoprophylaxis, the

* E. Saling, 'The Effect on the Foetus of Maternal Hyperventilation during Labour', *J. Obstet. Gynaec. Br. Emp.*, Vol. 76 (Oct. 1969).

psychophysical method and hypnosis—also tended to overbreathe.*
It is frequently socially dictated to the extent that the woman
breathes in and out to the accompaniment of hand-claps, drum-
beats, shouts, the reiterated name of God, her own cries for her
mother, or other exclamations, or according to instructions given by
a labour coach.

Overbreathing is so well-known to the experienced midwife that
she may watch a woman's respiration to gauge how far she is
advanced in labour. Untrained peasant midwives, or *nanas*, in
Jamaica, do this, and instruct women approaching full dilatation to
breathe shallowly and rapidly when they are 'too much hackling'.
This pattern of heavy, gasping breathing is not, however, confined
to childbirth. It may accompany strenuous physical work performed
over a short period of time and also religious worship involving
spirit possession and rebirth.

When I was engaged in an anthropological research of 'store-
front churches' in Chicago I participated in revivalist services and
watched worshippers going into trance-like states without fully
realizing what I was observing physiologically. I thought then that
this was a form of hysteria, and indeed, it may often be adequately
explained in these terms.† I was invited to preach to congregations
of Holy Rollers, and found that by reiterated spasmodic phrases and
exclamations in which the worshippers also joined I was able to
initiate the same ecstatic states, and that I too could lead participants
to be 'saved', who crumpled up and rolled in the aisles after sharing
in an ecstatic frenzy in which they gasped, swayed and jerked.

Only when I tape-recorded religious services in the hills in
Jamaica and then taped the cries and breathing rhythms of peasant
women in labour in the big public maternity hospital in Kingston,
did I realize that I was hearing the same kind of breathing associated
with almost identical utterances, and that in each case the breathing
was socially regulated by background cries, percussion instruments,
and Biblical recitation and chanting. I went back to the revivalist
services and the hospital with fresh eyes. Then I observed that dance-
like movements, particularly those involving pelvic rocking, also

* R. St. J. Buxton, 'Maternal Respiration in Labour', *I.A.C.P.* (1968).
† William Sargent, *The Battle of the Mind* (New York, Pan, 1900).

dictated the tempo and even the level of respiration, and that chant, physical movement and respiration were inextricably linked. In Jamaica this pattern is deliberately adopted in order to get the spirit and speak in tongues. It is called *labouring*.

Thus Jamaican peasants have incorporated overbreathing into revivalist religion: when they breathe repeatedly like this they are likely to experience tingling in the fingers, dizziness, peripheral anaesthesia, disorientation, hallucination and temporary loss of consciousness.

In childbirth this same heavy rapid breathing can also result in giddiness, peripheral anaesthesia (and forced hyperventilation has been used for this reason by anaesthetists wanting to reduce the amount of medication a patient under surgery needs), carpopedal spasm and loss of consciousness. All this would not much matter if the effect was only on the mother. But because the baby in utero is in a symbiotic relationship with its mother through the delicate neuro-chemical bond of the placental circulation, the fetus is affected, and can be affected even before the mother herself shows any symptoms of hyperventilation. With modern methods of analysing a drop of blood taken from the fetal scalp, blood chemistry changes resulting from hyperventilation or other causes can be detected early, and more precise measurement is possible than has ever existed before. The altiology of the physiological processes by which lack of balance between the carbon dioxide and oxygen in the maternal circulation can result in oxygen lack in the fetus, and the resulting changes in the pH factor in the fetal bloodstream, have been described.*

Breathing which at the same time is both deep and quick soon results, for most women, in a flushing-out of carbon dioxide from the maternal bloodstream, and a state of alkalosis or hypocapnea.

↑ in alkali reserve in blood

* An excellent summary of American and some British literature on the subject was written by Madeleine Shearer, in *Childbirth Education*, Vol. II, No. 4 (American Society for Psychoprophylaxis in Obstetrics, 1969). Also see J. Lumley and others, 'Hyperventilation in Obstetrics', *Am. J. Obstet. Gynec.* (March 1969); Wallace O. Fenn and Hermann Rahn, eds., *Handbook of Physiology, Section 3, Respiration*, Vol. I (Washington, D.C., American Physiological Society, 1965); and E. Saling, *J. Obstet. Gynaec. Br. Emp.*, Vol. 76 (Oct. 1969).

confirmed by est. of CO_2
treated by Na_3 or NH_3Cl
intravenously to ↑
excretion of bicarb.
by kidneys

The blood vessels passing through the placenta go into spasm, and the resulting constriction cuts down the blood flow to the baby. This can result, especially in a baby whose responsiveness to life is for other reasons limited, in the child being born limp and blue and in taking some time to breathe.

It is neither simply rapid breathing nor deep breathing which can do this. Overbreathing involves rapid deep breathing. This type of respiration can be abdominal or diaphragmatic-costal. It can also be what is often described as 'shallow-chest breathing' or 'third level' if there is a near-complete, gaseous exchange with each respiratory movement. This can occur, for example, when a woman blows out repeatedly, or when she cries out in pain or terror. The effect is intensified by muscular tension in the throat and shoulders and in the chest wall.

I have come to the conclusion that we ought to free ourselves from the mechanistic approach of teaching breathing in numbered levels and aim instead at helping each woman relate her breathing rhythms to the intensity and flow of each contraction, finding the level and rate that is right for her. It is more important to introduce exercises which promote rhythmic, easy, unforced breathing—whether it is slow or accelerated, deep or shallow—than it is to teach women how to do so many breaths per minute or so many a contraction. For whatever 'levels' are used in labour, breathing must be relaxed if hyperventilation is not to prove a problem. The approach which entails learning how to breathe to a count of 1–2–3–4–5–6, or whatever, is not, therefore, the best one.

It is perhaps particularly dangerous to teach a student breathing as a distraction technique which will help her shut off sensations from the uterus; the uterus is her *guide* and provides the physiological stimulus to which she is required to relate through her breathing. If a labour attendant dictates a breathing pattern which is not perfectly synchronized with the contraction the woman has become like an orchestra without a conductor.

It is only too easy under such circumstances to equip the woman in labour with all of the skills, but none of the art.

When I teach I instruct each woman once, and once only, in levels and rates of breathing for labour. This is a rudimentary exercise, a little as one might learn scales before proceeding to play the piano. The actual exercises are not those required for labour, and only give the basic technical equipment, which must then be built into the 'music' with which the breathing relates to contractions in labour.

The Stanislavsky acting method exercises, already described, can also be modified to teach *awareness of breathing*.* Thus (and I suggest they close their eyes for this one): 'You are in a dark country lane. It is the dead of night, there is no moon, everything is very still, except for the almost imperceptible movement of grasses and leaves. A twig snaps behind you. It was not your foot which trod on it! Somebody, something, is following you. . . .' Pupils feel themselves in the situation, and then discuss what happened to them, and what happened to their breathing.

Other imaginative exercises of this type can be highly pleasurable and provide a valuable contrast: 'You are lying on warm, sun-drenched sand, sun pouring down over your skin. You feel glowing with light and heat. There is blue haze of sea in front of you, sand firmly supporting your whole body. Everything is wrapped in silence. What is happening to your breathing?'. . . . 'You are smelling a richly scented rose cupped in your hands, great deep red petals. What happens to your breathing?'

In such exercises the breathing is a *by-product* of the imagined state and of what Stanislavsky called <u>emotion memory</u>. The teacher should avoid telling members of the group how to breathe as they act these scenes. The variations in breathing occur spontaneously, and only then are the actors asked to observe *how* they are breathing.

When a woman habitually breathes very shallowly I find it useful to teach some exercises in controlled slow, full breathing. Note, however, that one cannot meet a woman for the first time in late pregnancy, when the fundus is high, and tell whether a pattern of superficial breathing is a natural response to advanced pregnancy or an habitual breathing pattern.†

---

* Any teacher experimenting with this method might explore Flanders Dunbar, *Emotions and Bodily Changes* (New York, Columbia University Press, 1946), a basic and invaluable textbook on this subject.

† M. M. Garrey and Others, *Obstetrics Illustrated* (Edinburgh, Livingstone, 1969).

Women who breathe arrythmically, tightening their shoulders and sucking their breath in rapidly, can sometimes gain special insight into psychosomatic responses during antenatal preparation. Emphasis upon swinging the ribs out and on diaphragmatic breathing does not really help these women, since the result is often a strained, jerky movement of the diaphragm. They need to learn first how to let breathing flow right through them, and to associate it with pleasurable feelings in the abdomen and genital regions.

The teaching of a full, free, diaphragmatic breathing is best evolved from *relaxed abdominal* breathing, and there is still a need to teach abdominal breathing—but as involving 'here and now' awareness, rather than as a mechanical exercise. Each woman should be propped up well, with support right up the spine, and with her hands cupped over her lower abdomen. She is asked to breathe slowly and peacefully, feeling that the breath is flowing right down to where her hands are resting. She is encouraged to appreciate the feeling of her abdomen swelling out as she breathes in and subsiding as she breathes out. She takes the breath in through the nose, allowing the nostrils to dilate, and lets it flow out through a relaxed mouth, the lips soft and parted ('as if you have on a new, glossy and very expensive lipstick'). The teacher can describe the position of the baby inside the rocking cradle of the maternal pelvis, lapped in the waters of its private sea, sheltered in the darkness of her body. As the mother listens to the sound of her own breathing it is rather like waves washing on the shingle. This peaceful, slow deep breathing finds a place in teaching for between contractions in labour, to ensure that full use is made of the time between contractions, however short, to get complete refreshment.

It is only after teaching this type of breathing that I now instruct women in deep-chest, middle-chest, and shallow-chest breathing—patterns with which all readers should be familiar. I never put emphasis on forceful chest expansion, however, which often leads to strained breathing and, under stress, to overbreathing. Instead I find that breathing levels are best taught with emphasis on sensations at different levels *in the back* and with firm guiding hand pressure from a partner working with her at waist, upper waist and beneath the shoulder blades.

The lightest, quickest breathing I teach I call *mouth-centred* or *butterfly breathing*. If breathing is to be rapid it must at the same time be light, or hyperventilation may result. In labour, breathing almost invariably does become quicker as dilatation proceeds, whether the woman is instructed or completely untaught, whether she is having a difficult or easy labour, and whether it is her first or tenth child. This quicker breathing does not, in itself, spell panic or suffering.

This pattern of breathing is less pronounced and a good deal lighter than that sometimes called *panting* which was introduced first by Lamaze in France, then in Britain and the United States. The rationale for this breathing was that it reduced pressure on the uterus. Changes in intrauterine pressure as the result of different kinds of breathing are rarely observed, however,

Lightness can be encouraged by the use of verbal analogy: like a bubble on top of a wave . . . like a sparrow's feather . . . a humming bird drawing nectar from a flower . . . tissue paper in the breeze . . . a leaf on a birch tree . . . a balloon hanging by an open window patted against the wall by a breath of wind. . . . The similes must be appropriate for the culture and the individual woman concerned. Each teacher will need a variety to trigger off the requisite response in each student.

To keep the breathing comfortably light the muscles of the face, mouth and neck must be relaxed. Once a woman's head starts to be pressed back into the pillow, her face to fix itself like a mask, or her chin to be thrown up into the air, muscle tensions are involved which build up until she is panting heavily. So the teaching of breathing for labour cannot be divorced from the teaching of relaxation.

When giving support for labour, if a woman starts to drag through a difficult contraction, panting heavily and gasping at its height, breathe with her and coax her into lifting her breathing up and over the contraction like, for example, 'a hovercraft on a wave'.

In teaching mouth-centred breathing I always allow a margin for rather heavier breathing under the stress of the final processes of dilatation.

Once the rudimentary breathing techniques are learned these can be incorporated in a sensitivity response to contractions, using the pressure of the husband's hand on the upper leg to simulate a contraction. The husband pinches a small area of flesh on the inner thigh, holding it firmly grasped for forty-five to sixty seconds, and then releasing it by degrees. The key to her response is in the concept of a *wave*. Contractions are waves of pressure coming at varying but steadily decreasing intervals in an undulating rhythmic pattern; the crest of the wave is the height of the contraction. And, as with waves of the sea, each one contributes to the sweep forward of the incoming tide, which in this case is the birth of the baby. This concept of rhythmic flow, of a natural sweep of events, permits the student to integrate initially isolated techniques into a total pattern of psychosomatic adjustment to her labour, and it is this total pattern which is all-important. (The wave concept is not the only suitable one. In other societies and among people unfamiliar with or fearful of the sea, concepts of undulating hills and steep mountains may be more suitable.)

I explain the whole adjustment response necessary for breathing in the first stage of labour as *Wave Breathing*. As the wave rises the breathing becomes shallower and more rapid. It is important that the woman shall always be able to listen to the sound of her own breathing, so that her conscious appreciation of its rhythm prevents any possibility of it running away with her. An important element is *focused concentration* on breathing in harmony with internal activity. If at any point she feels she is losing the rhythm, tensing her throat muscles, or has the impression that her breath is being caught, she merely blows out crisply as if blowing out a birthday cake candle, and carries straight on. She is encouraged never to continue mouth-centred breathing desperately if she feels uncomfortable, but to blow in this way, and this easy blow out can then find a place within her breathing patterns as she proceeds through the late first stage and into the second.

It is in transition that hyperventilation is most likely to occur, because at this phase contractions tend to be more or less unpredictable, and the onset of the catch in the throat which heralds the expulsive reflex can only be adequately coped with by exhaling fast. As the urge builds up, becoming more and more imperative, the woman who is waiting for instructions before she feels free to push may find herself blowing out so frequently and heavily that there is a resulting carbon dioxide/oxygen inbalance. Especially is this so if she has been taught what some teachers call 'choo-choo breathing' or 'huffing and puffing,' which in some cases is also accompanied by bizarre, and at times frantic, activity, involving rocking the head from side to side, movements of the shoulders in a slump forward, or swinging of the arms. Such physical activity can itself encourage overbreathing, since it adds to the stress occasioned by the contractions an extra muscular activity which can lead to more energetic breathing. (Try doing any of these movements—for ten minutes only—in the exaggerated form in which they can be observed by a woman in labour who is reaching the end of her capacity for endurance, and one can soon see that breathing rhythms are quickly affected.)

In the second stage of labour a woman should be told to hold her breath just as long as she comfortably can, and no longer. I emphasize that the baby will be born with her breathing. She holds her breath no longer, and with no more sense of strain, than an opera singer reaching and holding a high note. It takes skill and control, but only those muscles which need to be used are contracted, and in this case the diaphragm alone is sufficient to help the strongly contracting uterus in its work. Once the head is on the perineum, and can be seen the size of an after-dinner coffee cup in the vagina at the height of each contraction, I suggest that the mother does only mouth-centred breathing, and no more deep breaths. In this way the head is breathed out more gently than when strong pushing continues to the point of crowning, and the mother reaches the fulfilment of her labour not like a sprinter crashing through the tape, but more like a boat being moored with precision and skill.

Husbands and Wives

15

The Father's Part in Labour

Katharine wrote in her labour report:

Our son finally put in an appearance yesterday morning. It was really 'child-birth with joy' and everything John and I had practised worked perfectly! I never once felt I was losing control, didn't get to the end my tether, re-mained very relaxed and had no desire for pethidine or gas and oxygen! I do hope this doesn't sound as though I'm blowing my own trumpet because the part I played in the whole thing was only equal to the parts played by John and the midwife.

The husband's presence can be used simply to encourage and give a sense of security to the woman. Or his role can be seen as primarily that of coaching, as a boxer's second coaches him in the ring. But teaching can go further than either of these and can involve him so completely that he participates with empathy in his wife's task in labour, and completes the course of classes with an understanding, tenderness and admiration for her greater than he ever had before. For this to happen he needs to be given an active role in classes, and to share fully in the relaxation and breathing exercises, and in discussion. He can himself learn how to relax, and what it means when his wife is really relaxed. He should be able to do the breathing himself, understand what problems are likely to crop up when her adaptive response to contractions is not perfect, and be able to carry her over difficult contractions by actually breathing with her, with-out at the same time tensing up or becoming anxious himself.

One of the first questions that men ask is how they can know the right time to take their wives to hospital, and many are anxious that any delay will lead to them having to do the delivery themselves. The teacher can say that when labour starts there is very rarely any immediate rush to get to hospital. A common pattern is for labour to start gradually, often over a matter of days, with contractions ten minutes apart and lasting less than a minute. The husband should be told that it is not only the frequency of contractions but their length and strength which is important, and contractions lasting less than a minute usually herald the beginning of labour, while they last a minute or more once labour is well under way.

Many women can sleep during early labour, and most comfortably in their own beds, or can go for a walk in the park or countryside, or to a film. The teacher may add that it is clear from the questions that they raise in classes, especially when they first attend, that men are nervous that they will be left delivering the baby, and that as a result many women are admitted to hospital when they still have a long labour in front of them. A woman will have learned in classes exactly how labour may start. She, too, may become excited and even apprehensive. The teacher can take the opportunity to say that it is up to her husband to keep calm, to make a careful note of all the signs of early labour, to encourage her to concentrate on other activities, and when it is useful help her to start doing her breathing and relaxation so that she is adjusting well to contractions and is handling her labour with a sense of purpose and achievement even before she goes into hospital.

Usually only when contractions are coming five minutes apart or less *and are lasting at least a minute* is it necessary to go to hospital, the only exceptions being when there is a good deal of bleeding (more than at the start of a period), when the waters go with a rush, or when the hospital has made it explicit that in her particular case they want her in as soon as there are signs of the beginning of labour.

The husband helps most who remains unflustered, and who is also able to maintain good relations with all members of staff whom the couple encounter during labour. It is not only fear, or pain, which can cause tension in his wife, but also frustration and a feeling that others may disapprove of what she is trying to do. So his tact, good humour and ability to explain what his wife is aiming at doing in labour can all ease her path and make her labour more comfortable. He should go into hospital realizing that the primary concern of midwives and doctors is to ensure the physical health of mother and baby, and not the psychological welfare of the family.

Occasionally a member of staff will feel that a husband has come in to try and 'take over', and it is up to him by his own understanding of their roles to convince them that his presence is helpful. In the modern hospital there is always something to be learned, and usually members of staff are willing to explain devices such as monitoring equipment and the many other machines which now regulate and record labour, subjects of fascinating interests to many husbands, and often also to the woman in labour.

But however many machines there are ticking away, the most important person in the labour room is the woman having the baby. It is easy to forget this and when a woman is linked to a fetal heart monitor to look at the screen recording the contraction rather than at the woman herself. Eye-to-eye contact, and for a large part of labour for most women, body contact, in the form of gentle stroking or firm holding can be very supportive during each contraction. When a contraction starts the man should stop talking and concentrate on giving support to his wife, however pretty the midwife, or however fascinating the obstetrics being explained to him!

When the woman comes to the end of the first stage, with contractions coming every two minutes or even less, and lasting a minute or more, she often does not want to be touched at all. A perceptive husband realizes this. It is a sign of progress. Some women like to sit more upright, feeling the baby's head pressing right down against the anus and vagina, but it is a time when it is extremely difficult to adjust one's position, as it is a bit like sitting on a large grapefruit. In the class not only the woman, but her husband too, can try what it feels like to sit with a shoe just underneath the buttocks approximately in the position of the baby's head as it presses against the rectum and anus. In labour he can help by shifting his wife into a more comfortable position, well propped up with five or six pillows, and if necessary his arm too.

It also helps to see that the woman's mouth does not get dry, especially when she is breathing through her parted lips. This can be ensured by giving her sips of water or ice chips to suck (the teacher can mention that it is a good idea to take some ice in in a thermos), or to let her suck on a sponge with which the husband freshens up her face between contractions (a small, new cosmetic sponge is best for this), and a lip gloss or petroleum jelly will help to avoid her lips becoming dry. A woman who is doing little light mouth-centred breaths over the tops of difficult contractions may find that it helps if occasionally she breathes with the tip of her tongue raised and lightly pressed against the hard palate behind her front top teeth, as her mouth will then remain moist.

Another thing which most husbands are very good at is massage. The antenatal teacher can explain that basically pain or aching can be in two main places, over the uterus itself, and especially over the cervix, which is the part which is opening, and in the low small of the back, where the pelvis joins the spine. The cervix projects into the vagina like the stem of a bottle, and during the first stage of labour it is first of all drawn up and thinned out so that it becomes one with the main body of the uterus, and then begins to open wider and wider. This process is called *dilatation* and the progress of the whole first stage is measured in terms of dilatation.

The stretching of the cervix can cause pain, which often radiates out into the groin and sometimes down the thighs, which may cause a feeling of pulling against the pubic bone at the front (since the baby's head is probably being pressed down towards it), and may also spread right round to the back, rather as if a wide band of elastic were being pulled tighter and tighter. At the peak of the contraction the pull feels greatest, and then it starts to fade away again, each contraction lasting about one minute.

Light abdominal massage over the very bottom of the bulge where the baby's head usually is can be very comforting. But it must be light. The husband strokes 'as if stroking the baby's head' with his wrist lifted, using a movement similar to that when touching velvet or any soft fabric. This is often helpful during contractions. The men practise this light abdominal massage in class, and the teacher goes round to help, advise and give approval.

If there is pain both in the front and in the back the hospital may

be happy for her to have a hot water bottle against the lower spine—
a baby's hot water bottle is ideal. Sometimes there are rules that these
are not allowed in case they leak, so it is a good idea to take in a
picnic freezing pack which he has boiled up in a saucepan of water
and wrapped in a few layers of aluminium foil to keep hot. These
can easily be reheated as there is always hot water available in the
hospital.

If, however, pain is concentrated in the back it is usually better for
the wife to lie on her side, whichever side is most comfortable, and
her husband uses firm pressure with the heel of his palm against the
part which is hurting, which is the area directly over the sacrum,
against which the baby's head is pressing as it passes through the
pelvis. This can be varied with firm circular massage, moving
the flesh on the bone, and every now and again sweeping out over the
sides of the buttocks. Here again the men experiment with different
kinds of back massage in class, and find out what their wives like.
If the husband is getting tired of back rubbing and wants a break he
can sit so that his own hip is pressed against this sacrolumbar region,
leaning back slightly so that his own body weight provides firm
support for his wife's back. It is worth practising all these techniques
well in advance and rehearsing them frequently so that there need be
no fumbling and confusion when labour starts.

Many women become more or less disoriented in labour, especially towards the end of the first stage, and particularly if they have
had pain relieving drugs which tend to make them slightly drunk.
Some women do not mind this, but perhaps most of them try to get
a grip on things, and this causes tension. Some assistance in recollect-
ing the pattern of the labour and the progress that has been made,
and help in coping with each contraction as it comes, is essential. It is
useful for the husband and wife together to keep a log book in which
they write down in one column what is happening, in the next the
adaptive techniques the woman is using in responding to this, and in
the next anything that is being done to help her by her husband or
other attendants at this point, including things which are said. In this
way neither one will feel that they are losing their bearings in
labour.

Even while they are still at home they can record how often

contractions are coming and how long they are lasting, as this is important information to have at one's fingertips when they ring the hospital to say they think labour has started. They can also note when she empties her bladder, as it is a good idea to do this every hour or so to avoid urine building up and so both causing a pressure pain and delaying the descent of the baby's head.

If the woman is getting drowsy or tired it helps to reassure that it is perfectly all right to drop off to sleep in between contractions, and the husband will wake her as the contraction starts so that she can breathe her way over it. They come so regularly that he can tell when another is due from his watch, especially if he has been recording the pattern of contractions. He can also place a hand gently on her uterus to feel as it is beginning to go hard. The teacher can explain that it feels rather as if one's hand was on a balloon which was being blown up. The watch is also useful to tell the labouring woman the phase of the contraction reached. Thus he can break contractions down into ten-second stretches, counting them off for her, or he can say 'a third of the way through now' . . . 'halfway' . . . 'two-thirds' . . . or simply count slowly. Some women love this, and others find it irritating. Find out which techniques suit each woman. But every woman needs encouragement, especially as she enters what often feels like a stormy sea of labour near full dilatation of the cervix. A man can never go wrong by giving her praise and saying Good or Splendid or whatever seems right as she goes over the wave of the contraction.

As soon as teachers start to talk about the second stage they will discover that many men, especially early on in the course before they have heard a range of labour reports from other husbands, expect to withdraw at this point and hand over to experts, and that although fewer and fewer men plan actually to leave the room and wait outside while the baby is delivered, many others see their role as passive, and although they want to watch the birth, do not anticipate actually being able to help at this stage. So it may be a good idea to ask a couples' class or fathers' evening 'What do you envisage yourself doing to help your wife in the second stage? Is there any way you think you can help her?' and to explore the various ways in which loving support can be given then.

Probably most antenatal teachers nowadays believe that the husband's presence in the second stage is not primarily so that he can be a witness to the delivery of his child, but that he can share the experience through which his wife is passing and can give her encouragement, guidance, physical support, and love. It is then particularly that he can serve as an interpreter between midwives or doctors and his wife, as well as being the reassuring, reliable friend who is there even though bells ring, figures in white or green flood into the room, though alarming trays of instruments may be rolled up to the end of the delivery table, and although she may suddenly find that the lower half of her body has been taken over by strangers and somehow appropriated by the hospital. This can happen even when things are going well. How much more necessary is his support when matters are not so straightforward!

There is a case to be made for each man to make an appointment to meet his wife's obstetrician so that they can discuss the management of the labour and delivery and he can find out whether he can stay with her whatever happens, if she wishes him to be present. He will often be told that if a forceps delivery is necessary, for example, he must leave, and indeed he has no legal right to insist on being there. But at least he will have been able to help his wife for as long as he could, and will also have made his point that he would like to remain—in itself an act which, provided enough men do it, will gradually erode opposition, although it may take years to do so.

The husband's place in the second stage is at the head end, not in a corner gazing at the perineal view of delivery. Exciting as it can be to lean forward to see exactly what is happening on the perineum, the woman needs his physical touch and his concentrated attention on her as a person, and not simply on her dilating vulva. So he can stand or sit at her side, with his arm around her head and shoulders so that she is propped well up, and as a firm basis from which to push. With five or six pillows, he can cradle one over his forearm, so providing a wider supporting area immediately behind her neck and shoulders, although it is important that she can raise her head easily to take a deep breath, without feeling that her head is being forced forward on her chest. The closer he can get to her, the better. This is partly so that *he* does not get backache. If he is allowed to sit on the bed or on a stool very near his wife his own shoulder can add to the support he can give her. With many delivery tables he will need to watch to see that pillows do not slip between the bars at the head of the table, and every now and again, between contractions, may need to plump them up and see that they really are allowing his wife's trunk to be raised to a good angle for bearing down.

Many teachers suggest that the husband should reinforce the encouragement to push which is often offered by obstetricians and midwives. I feel that this is out of place and only encourages the woman to strain. The appropriate phrase for the husband to use is 'open up'. This is where it can be useful to discuss with husbands the material on the second stage which is in the section 'The Skills We Teach'.

The woman may welcome sips of water, having her face washed or refreshed with an ice cold damp sponge, or a hot or cold face flannel, and having her hair brushed back and up and away from the nape of her neck. The husband can hold a small mirror angled over her abdomen so that she can see the top of the baby's head once it is visible in the birth canal, but this needs practice in bed beforehand, or he may get the angle wrong, especially if he is excited. He should be quick to notice if she gets cramp, and to rub the affected area. Cramp almost invariably occurs in muscles which are not relaxed, so it is important that he helps her to relax her legs, so that she does not push through them.

When the instruction is given to stop pushing, or to pant, or even to go gently, or some similar command, he can tell her to breathe and can breathe *with* her, jaw dropped, mouth relaxed, concentrating on the breath *out* to echo the sense of the baby slipping forward and out. He must realize that ideally the baby is *breathed* out, and not pushed out.

All this is a matter also of working out with whoever is doing the delivery what is best in the circumstances, and the essence of this is communication. Discussion should always take place between contractions, never during them, when his attention should be on his wife.

Because I always arrange for couples who have recently had babies to return to classes to tell of their experiences, by the end of every course pupils will have heard what husbands did and how they reacted, not once, but probably many times. The new parents come towards the end of the class, and they often come in with the baby in a carrier strapped to the husband, and nestled against his chest, or in a carry-cot which he is holding.

As the wife starts to tell the story of her labour and the husband cuddles his baby, shared responsibility in parenthood comes over very clearly. This can be an important experience for the man who feels that for a man to be interested in a small baby is effeminate and emasculating, and that it is 'soft' to like to stroke and kiss and talk nonsense to a two-week-old infant. I ask the wife, 'What did your husband do that helped you?' and also enquire of him 'What did you find helped her most?' Many of the techniques of support I myself use and teach I have learned from couples I have taught.

In a couples' class or fathers' evening the teacher can also ask the husband, 'Have you any tips for the other men here?' and 'Is there anything you didn't learn or didn't remember which you wish that you had?' Both questions which can lead to good discussion. Do not gloss over errors of judgement or omissions in teaching: learn from the experience. We should avoid painting a fantasy picture of an ideal labour to which all the other couples feel they ought to live up, rather face reality, with all that we can learn from it, and with the fascinating variety of human behaviour it presents.

Many couples describe an experience of profound joy, of intense wonder and delight, and frequently of something which I can only call ecstasy. I have learned that it is wise to ask the husband how he felt *after* the birth, when he had left his wife in hospital, when he had made all the telephone calls, and faced the empty bed and the untidy kitchen and the silence of the house or flat, because I now realize that when a husband has participated fully in the birth, and especially if he has been really 'high', there is bound to be an emotional drop afterwards. It is then, separated from his wife and very often alone, that he experiences his own kind of postnatal depression. If a man has friends or parents who share his excitement and the thrill of the delivery, and are approving of the role he played, this may not occur, but many men are treated as being slightly odd to get that much involved and meet with blank stares of non-comprehension or amused smiles. Just as a woman can feel she is empty once her baby is outside her, and especially so if it is not able to be close to her and in her arms whenever she wants to hold it, so a man can feel isolated and empty when he leaves his wife to be cared for by strangers in hospital.

One husband had been very close to his wife throughout a long and difficult labour during which she had depended on him utterly, went home and wandered aimlessly from room to room, and then rang me in tears as he tried to cope with the overwhelming sadness he felt from being deprived of both his wife and his newborn son. So this is another subject which should be discussed in any class when there are husbands present, and especially when new fathers can be there to tell of their own feelings and how they handled them. In concentrating all our attention on the mother's needs it is easy to forget that the new father is a parent too, and that when childbirth has been a joint endeavour there may be special emotional stresses immediately after. The exception to this is whenever a baby is born at home. Then birth is part of the continuum of normal daily living and the husband retains his responsibility for his wife and child. I believe that birth at home can make a significant contribution to the mental health of the family.

Wherever a couple choose or are advised to have their baby, it is a pity if the teacher stops short with discussing the husband's techniques of coaching a woman through her labour, and there should always be ample time for setting this in the context of the man's feelings about the birth. With this can come increased understanding for both man and woman of themselves and of each other.

16

Sex during Pregnancy
and in the Puerperium

The taboo on intercourse during all or part of pregnancy and in the immediate postnatal period varies enormously between different societies and even within societies, between different social classes or religious faiths, for instance. But certain common themes relating to pollution and purity emerge. The Judaeo-Christian cultural tradition—among many others—puts great emphasis on physical completeness, conceptualizing the human body as a container, the exits and entrances of which should normally be kept closed except on special, socially permitted occasions. We can see how in pregnancy the woman obviously has been penetrated and entered, and how after childbirth her body is still partially open. She is 'unclean' and therefore set apart.

Physical excretions—matter issuing from the margins of the body and the points of exit and entry—are envisaged as threatening also, either because they are considered disgusting in themselves or as causing illness to others. Thus in many societies faeces, urine, pus, blood, whether from a wound or resulting from menstruation or birth, semen, nasal mucus, sweat, saliva and even breast milk are seen as dangerous, polluting, and in certain specified circumstances as having magical powers. The postnatal taboo on coitus here relates also to the production of body substances which are thought to be contaminating. Menstrual blood or lochia may threaten the man's virility, or the male ejaculate may be considered a danger to the health or life of the new baby.

The woman, in both pregnancy and the puerperium, is passing through a transitional social state. She stands, as it were, on the margins of society, being neither one thing nor the other, but waiting to take a new role and social status. The baby, too, is in a state of becoming, not yet a member of society, not yet fitted into the pattern. Every society is concerned to order, classify and control relationships between its members. Marginal beings have no real identity. Both mother and child are in a state of ritual danger, vulnerable and exposed themselves, but frequently also bringing a risk to others.

A whole system of taboos and prohibitions, dietary regulations and other injunctions concerning conduct exist in societies throughout the world to cope with this situation, relating not only to the mother and baby but to the father of the child, and frequently also to other members of society coming into contact with them. Together these form the *rites de passage* which van Gennep saw as characteristic of transitional states of existence all over the world. One of the commonest of these concerns avoidance and separation. Sexual intercourse is the most intimate form of human contact, and as such is the epitome of proscribed relationships. This applies not only to childbirth but also to any undertaking involving explicit challenge or danger. Thus frequently sexual abstinence is enjoined before such diverse activities as battle, hunting wild animals, tapping palm wine, planting ground nuts, fishing, making pottery, or divination and religious observance.

Prohibitions on intercourse during pregnancy and in the puerperium in our own society are part of these larger culturally widespread and converging—and perhaps interconnected—taboo systems relating to marginal states, transitional rituals and body substances and orifices. Feelings of uncertainty, or of distaste, are shared not only by some prospective and new parents but by some doctors. There is even one book, published by a reputable American publisher, in which the author claims intercourse during pregnancy as the Original Sin, the physical effect of which is to cause malformed and brain-damaged babies.

Recent studies of the effect of prostaglandins on the muscle fibres of the uterus have led some to feel that doubts about the advisability of intercourse during pregnancy are confirmed, and this might be so until one remembers that the healthy uterus, pregnant or nonpregnant, contracts regularly—that it is a dynamic muscular organ and not merely a passive bag. The frequency of Braxton-Hicks contractions in late pregnancy indicates that contractions preparatory to labour are normal, whether or not they are associated with sexual arousal and with female orgasm or simply with the ejaculation of semen. If contractions prove strong and persistent and there is post-coital bleeding, this is an obvious contraindication to intercourse during pregnancy. Most couples, however, can have intercourse without such drastic effects.

The couple expecting a baby are not only prospective parents but also husband and wife and have a right to a sexual identity over and above their roles as father and mother. The concept of parenthood divorced from sex, of the virgin birth and various forms of extragenital fecundation run as themes through many different mythologies and examples abound in Buddhist, Graeco-Roman and Judaeo-Christian literature. They are psychologically enticing if only because the child wants to possess its parents completely. In infantile fantasy the ideal mother is the madonna figure who knows nothing of sexuality and gives herself utterly to her children. (The shadow side of this all-giving, all-good mother is the witch.)

As a result of these intermingling strands of socially reinforced myth and fantasy concerning primary bonds many couples feel guilty when they have intercourse during pregnancy, fearing that they are in some way harming the fetus or risking miscarriage or premature birth. I find that questions about whether it is all right to make love often arise towards the end of the first interview with the couples, sometimes after obviously less pressing matters have been fully discussed, when the subject is raised almost in the nature of an afterthought, or as they rise to leave, 'By the way, there's one more thing. . . .'

It is a topic which the expectant mother may want to discuss with her general practitioner obstetrician or with a marriage counsellor, but one which is only likely to arise when the counsellor can provide a comfortable opportunity and a relaxed, unhurried and receptive atmosphere. Not all couples will require guidance, nor should counselling ever be obtrusive, interfering or directive.

The perceptive doctor will observe when extra help or reassurance may be needed, and if he is sensitive to nuances in the relationships of couples he is treating may also be aware of the occasions when they are unable to ask for advice or to verbalize their anxieties. Such are the age, educational and social-class barriers between many doctors and their patients that some patients feel that they cannot talk about such subjects to a doctor in words suitable for, decent enough or intelligible to his ears. It is not always enough to wait till questions are asked by patients; to do so is to do what many parents do in a similar situation regarding imparting sexual information to their children: 'I will answer questions truthfully when he/she asks them.' But the children, aware of what is likely to prove embarrassing for all concerned, all too often tactfully avoid asking the questions. The doctor may have to open the door for discussion of the subject by asking whether a woman is feeling any different emotionally now that she is pregnant, how she feels about fetal movements and whether she likes or dislikes them, if she knows how the baby grows inside her and how it is protected in her uterus, or by introducing the subject of her feelings about her pregnancy in any way which seems appropriate for that particular patient. When there has been anxiety about conception or about holding on to the pregnancy, it may be wise during the second trimester for the doctor to ask casually whether they feel happy about making love again now, thus giving tacit approval, and indicating his willingness to listen if problems are being faced.

Women's feelings about intercourse in pregnancy are probably just as important as straight medical fact, and if a woman finds intercourse distasteful in late pregnancy, or during menstruation, persuading her that she should be able to take a more rational view, and that this taboo is just a remnant of dark myths rooted in prehistory is not only unlikely to be very successful but may do positive harm. The first rule is to respect each woman's personality and each couple's own inclinations in this respect.

Women may consult the antenatal teacher because they are worried about causing miscarriage or stillbirth. They may even feel rather ashamed that they want to have intercourse, believing that it is disapproved of by their professional advisers—doctors, nurses and midwives—since intercourse in pregnancy is rarely discussed in the antenatal clinic except in terms of avoiding sex when the pregnancy appears to be at risk. This is a pity, because a purely negative attitude to intercourse fails to recognize the positive surge of happiness and wonder that many couples feel when the pregnancy is confirmed. The antenatal teacher can be supportive and reassuring about sex in pregnancy.

Counselling need not be an invasion of privacy. All that is required is that the antenatal teacher, midwife or other counsellor is aware of the stresses through which the couple may be passing, takes it for granted that a happy couple make love, and, if there seems to be any nervousness about the safety of the unborn baby on the mother's or father's part, is able to refer explicitly and clearly to the manner in which the fetus is protected in its intrauterine environment and to ways in which intercourse can be suitably adapted to pregnancy.

Whenever there has been a long period of infertility, or a previous abortion, a woman is liable to feel herself reproductively inadequate, and one can assume that there is anxiety on this score. The antenatal teacher who encourages free discussion and sharing of hopes and problems in classes may often find this subject cropping up spontaneously and should be ready to comment in a helpful way, and to gently lead group participants to express their worries, if they wish to, and to give accurate information.

Worries range from concern that semen is contaminating and produces germs which can deform the baby, and the idea that the erect penis can penetrate the membranes and cause miscarriage and stillbirth, to anxiety that pressure on the abdomen may result in a flattened or otherwise damaged baby. Sometimes a man becomes impotent in pregnancy, at least with his wife, because he finds fetal movements threatening—'there is someone else there'—or the state of pregnancy disgusting and intercourse almost an incestuous act with a woman who now symbolises a mother. In these cases counselling should be done by a psychotherapist or other person who understands some of the deep unconscious factors involved.

Late in pregnancy women often find intercourse in the ventro-ventral position very uncomfortable. So it may be as well if the teacher mentions during classes that pressure on the abdomen during intercourse may make a woman feel acutely uncomfortable, that pressure on breasts may also be painful and result in leaking of colostrum, and that a couple can take pregnancy not only as a time to experiment with different positions but as an opportunity to explore other ways of making love. I always recommend the use of a good many pillows as an addition to comfort and pleasure during pregnancy and the puerperium. It depends entirely on the nature of the group as to whether more information is likely to be sought then and there, or information and opinions exchanged.

If discussion on this theme does develop in the group, the teacher can point out that even the ventroventral position can be satisfactory when the man kneels above his wife, keeping his weight off her body and supporting himself with his forearms. Coital postures in which the man penetrates from behind the woman, or in which she lies on her back or side with her legs swung across his thighs, are, however, generally preferable. This sort of position is particularly useful if the woman finds herself slow to reach orgasm, when the ability to move relatively freely so that she can achieve maximum stimulation, and not to be simply a passive partner, may be very important. Positions in which the woman kneels in front of or astride the man, avoiding pressure on abdomen and breasts, are also satisfactory methods of coitus for some women.

Once the fetus has engaged deep penetration may be painful, and it is wiser for her husband to introduce only the tip of the penis. The angle and depth of penetration from behind the woman can then be controlled by contraction of her glutei, and if she is reluctant herself to embark on the rhythmic movements leading to orgasm she can provide maximum stimulation for him by contraction and release of the glutei, pelvic rocking and pelvic-floor contractions. This is one of the ways in which expectant mothers can discover that learning body awareness and control in pregnancy results in skills applicable not only to pregnancy and labour but to intercourse.

Most books on sex advise the man to delay ejaculation until the woman is obviously embarked on the rhythmic movements immediately preceding orgasm. Although this may be wise normally, in the last trimester of pregnancy she may feel the erect penis as threatening and may be much better able to reach her climax immediately *after* he has ejaculated, when he is slightly detumescent, and consequently there is more room, and additional lubrication is provided by semen in the vagina.

If intercourse takes place with loving gentleness and tenderness many, probably most, women can enjoy love-making right through pregnancy and until labour starts. But in spite of this, many women go through a period during a pregnancy when they do not seem able to give both to a man and to the baby inside them—and the same feeling can exist during the puerperium, when it can be a cause of real marital tension.

A few women get strong uterine contractions during orgasm. Each woman will know if this is so with her. Nearly always they die down and disappear altogether if she lies quietly, perhaps with a hot water bottle against her abdomen or in the small of her back to help her relax. Occasionally, however, labour is initiated. Many couples use intercourse as a way of inducing labour which everyone was ready and waiting for. In some societies intercourse just before the onset and during the early first stage of labour is thought to be highly efficacious and to ensure a speedy and safe birth.

After the Birth

In the United States obstetricians usually say No for six or eight weeks before and after delivery. In France it is three weeks. In Britain obstetricians tend to say not until the first postnatal examination. If a woman has discomfort or pain on intercourse, however, it is of value if she is able to tell her obstetrician about this at her postnatal check-up.

There seems, however, to be no reason why a couple should not make love just whenever they are ready to. This is unlikely to be until the period of bloody discharge is over—say three or four days (or longer)—but after that a great many couples feel especially tender towards each other, and perhaps this happens particularly when the husband has shared in the birth.

Women who have had episiotomies or lacerations with subsequent suturing are unlikely to feel that they want intercourse for longer, and may feel very tender for months after; this depends on the extent and depth of the suturing and the skill with which it was done.* A woman can feel quite desperate then: Shall I never be 'myself' again? What is going to happen to us? She may wish to seek gynaecological help. Most women are physiologically ready for intercourse a week to ten days after delivery.† Yet even when a couple feel drawn together in this way it is clear that a great many women suffer entrance dyspareunia within the months after delivery which may persist as long as a year. Although this may be due to bad suturing of the perineum, sometimes although the suturing was efficiently done the management of labour was uncaring and unfriendly, and the woman suffered shock which created a mental association between delivery and rape. Often nervousness, ignorance and poor sexual technique result in the well-known postnatal secondary frigidity.

However pain-free the episiotomy and suturing, a woman may feel damaged, worries that she is not as she was before, and has fantasies about being 'in shreds down there'. Scar tissue often feels much more extensive than it is. Many women are reluctant to look in a mirror or even to touch themselves, partly because it is not 'nice' and partly because they are frightened of what they might find. Where delivery has been traumatic and the woman has fantasized it as a sort of rape these feelings may be carried over into intercourse. In such circumstances secondary frigidity is not an uncommon experience, with spasm of the levators, lack of lubrication and acute entrance dyspareunia.

After childbirth and after the period of normal vaginal discharge is over, natural secretions may be absent for some time. This means that although she can mentally and readily agree to the prospect of intercourse, a woman somehow cannot take her body with her, and there is no vaginal lubrication. She feels tight, dry, tender and unre-

---

* Sheila Kitzinger, ed., *Episiotomy, Physical and Emotional Aspects* (London, National Childbirth Trust, 1972).

†See W. H. Masters and V. E. Johnson, *Human Sexual Response* and *Human Sexual Inadequacy* (Boston, Little, Brown, 1966; 1970 respectively).

ceptive. Couples should not hesitate to use additional aids then. Whatever lubrication is used, however, it should not sting. They should try oil, any contraceptive cream, or a lubricating jelly instead.

The husband should use clitoral stimulation at this time so that his wife can be swept along on the same wave of passion as he is. Most authorities emphasize the desirability of complete and lengthy clitoral stimulation, and a man who is afraid of hurting his wife may concentrate on this to the exclusion of other, more effective sexual techniques. He may need to be reminded that there are many erogenous zones, and that in skilled and loving hands *any part* of a woman's (or a man's) body can become an erogenous zone. Clitoral stimulation should always include and indeed concentrate on the *shaft* of the clitoris, not its tip, and should not be persisted with once the clitoris is firm and swollen; if it is, the result can be intense irritation and even a feeling of desperation on the woman's part. Once the clitoris is clearly fully responsive to stimulation it is time for gentle penetration.

As the man penetrates he should avoid pressure on the site of the episiotomy. It is quite simple to explain to a couple exactly where this is. Using pillows under the woman so that she is tilted at the correct angle, he can enter so that pressure is directed forwards, towards the clitoris. If the woman is sufficiently stimulated, the vagina, however small before, will have become dilated and tentlike. In this way a woman with a rather tight vagina can easily contain the erect penis, *provided she is aroused*.

Some couples find that loss of pelvic-floor tone as a result of pregnancy and labour leads to less satisfying intercourse after the baby comes, the problem being that the vagina is slack and inadequate to grip the penis. A great deal can be done by regular exercise of the muscles not only at exercise sessions but at times recurring throughout the day—whenever the mother changes a nappy, goes up or down stairs, stands waiting for a bus or train or to be served in a shop, when she cooks, washes the dishes, or feeds the baby. Such pelvic-floor movements should always finish with a pulling-in contraction—never a flop and sag. The vaginal kiss in coitus is itself an excellent way of increasing the tone of the levator muscles.

Doctors are unwilling to fit a vaginal diaphragm or an IUD for two or three months, or sometimes even longer, after delivery. Breastfeeding mothers should not take the contraceptive pill at least until lactation is well established, and then the 'mini' pill seems the best. Moreover, a sheath used by the man is the method of contraception least likely to be aesthetically acceptable after childbirth; unless a good deal of lubricating cream or a ready lubricated sheath is used it can also be painful. Although a sheath can be satisfactory, if it is not, the answer is probably either to use a previously prescribed contraceptive cap, which probably *will not fit properly*, but will, if used with plenty of contraceptive cream, be extremely unlikely to result in pregnancy, or to use Emko foam with the applicator.

A woman cannot conceive until she has ovulated. But she may ovulate a couple of weeks before she gets her first period after having a baby. So there is no way of knowing when she may be fertile again. She is less likely to ovulate while she is breast feeding, but cannot rely upon that.

In talking to expectant mothers about these matters it is far better to introduce the subjects casually as they seem relevant at various points during the course than to start a lecture on sex which many may find difficult to take in one undigested lump. The teacher must respect the pupils' religious and moral convictions and, perhaps, prejudices. Sometimes the obvious and natural place for discussion of some of these matters is with the couple during a private interview, and this is especially so if there are any real problems, but if you undertake this you must be sensitive to the couple's needs and use a very cautious approach, avoiding a doctrinaire attitude on the one hand and embarrassed facetiousness on the other. In fact, one has to get to know people as individuals first of all, and then it all seems to fall into place. Not all couples require guidance of this kind, but the perceptive counsellor will be sensitively aware to observe when extra help is needed. Childbirth can be an important growing point in a couple's relationship, and childbirth educators can help this process by seeing pregnancy and birth within the context of the marriage.

Birth

17

Support in Labour

If you are giving support in labour to your own pupils you will already know each other, and there should be few problems. But if you are required to help someone with no previous instruction some techniques may be useful which I developed when working with clinic patients in Latin America and the West Indies. Often these women were already distressed when we met, and the initial problem was that of getting them to stop screaming so that they could notice that there was somebody there trying to help them.

In Germany 'a bath course' is sometimes given to women who have received no previous instruction. A nurse prepares the patient and then goes with her into the bathroom, where she sits and teaches her how to relax and breathe for labour and explains what will happen, whilst she is in the peaceful atmosphere of the bath.

Many of these suggestions may also be helpful with women who have attended classes, and can form the basis of instruction when a husband is acting as labour coach for his wife.

If you are not already on the staff it is important to learn the hospital routines and names of staff where possible. Try to discover which hospital procedures are inflexible and which can be altered in individual cases or under certain circumstances. If, as in many American hospitals, liquids by mouth are never allowed during labour—a practice which can be the cause of great misery to a woman in hard labour, especially in hot weather—the mother may still be permitted to have her lips moistened with a sponge on which she can suck, and iced water may be available for this purpose. In the absence of a sponge, a strip of gauze, or even paper towels, will do.

Wear very light-weight clothing. This is hot, sticky and tiring work, and you will be in close physical contact with the mother.

Get as nearly as possible at the same level as the labouring woman; do not tower over her. So sit on a chair by the bed where she can see you easily. Until she has understood some simple breathing techniques, only instruct *between* contractions. Later you will be able to encourage and praise her during contractions.

Introduce yourself clearly. Say if you have children and how many. Your role is not so much that of teacher or even mother—and certainly not that of drill sergeant—as it is that of a *sister* who understands what she is feeling and knows what to do about it. Speak quietly and gently, but with firmness and confidence, and smile. This applies to the second as well as the first stage. Everything you say should have positive value in helping her. The French call it *verbal asepsis*, but it is not only a question of not introducing negative elements, but of giving the support that means that every phrase is an emotional cocktail for the woman. If she is still in early labour, have some general conversation in which you get to know each other. If you can do so, compliment her on her nightdress or hair, or anything else which helps her feel more of a person, and less of a patient.

Help her get into a comfortable position in which she is not lying flat staring up at white tiles or ceiling. Prop her well, raising the bed-head if possible, and see she has good support right up her spine so that she can relax better. The very change of posture may help her get off to a fresh start. Sometimes a woman will be allowed up out of bed, and you can stroll around with her as you talk. This will help the presenting part to descend and press against the cervix, so it can be obstetrically, as well as emotionally, useful.

If she is hot sponge her face with a sponge or cloth and cold, preferably iced, water, or wipe her face with a flannel wrung out in warm water. Brush her hair back from her face and up from the nape of the neck, and if it is long, tie it with ribbons or a gauze strip.

Clean her spectacles for her if they have misted over and, indeed, ensure that she can see throughout labour.

Offer her a sip of iced water.

If she is moaning or weeping, wait patiently till it decreases as a contraction finishes, and then ask, 'Has it finished? . . . Then rest now, and I will help you.' Tell her that she can learn how to work with her body and with her womb which you know is tightening hard. Of course it hurts. (Never deny pain.) But it will hurt less when she knows what to do.

'The tightenings of the womb come and go, don't they? They are like waves'—or mountains (depending on cultural background). Describe as suggested for classes. 'Rest completely between each one and you will have strength for the next one. When the end of the next one comes I want you to blow out—a long, long blow out, like this . . . through your mouth, to mark the end of it. Then you will feel fresh, and I can help you in the rest time.'

You have now established the difference between a contraction and not having a contraction. It may sound rather obvious, but it is a distinction of which the woman in a panic of fear and pain may be oblivious. The distinction will, in itself, help her not to get exhausted. The exhausted woman can learn very little, and cannot summon up the energy for adaptive techniques of the kind which she needs in labour.

Do *not* tell her to 'relax'. It is useless to talk to a woman who has never learned neuromuscular control to relax in a situation of stress such as that at the end of the first stage of labour. It will only irritate and confuse her further. Concentrate on her breathing instead. Suggest that she meets each contraction (using whatever term seems best in order to get her understanding cooperation) with very slow breathing. If she is less than 6 or 7 centimetres dilated she may be able to get through the contraction with slow breathing alone if you breathe with her. If she seems to have withdrawn into a nightmare world of her own she may not even be aware, however, that you are breathing with her.

Regulate her breathing with a relaxed hand, stroking her arm from shoulder down to hand as a tactile signal for each expiration. Once reassured in this way, and finding that a contraction is easier when she breathes slowly, she will probably open her eyes, and then you can say 'I will breathe with you. Watch me and we will do this together.' If using the term *contraction* try to know what this means for the labouring woman; amongst West Indians, for instance, a contraction means 'cramp', often acutely painful, so for them it is a very unsuitable term, and *the womb tightening* is better.

If there is stress and she is more than 5 centimetres dilated, it is likely that she will need to breathe more shallowly and rapidly over the peaks. So just *before* the point when she looks as if she is going to be submerged by pain, tell her to breathe quickly and lightly through her parted lips. She will probably throw back her head, contracting muscles in neck and shoulders and start to moan or cry. Tell her firmly to open her eyes and look at you: 'Watch my hand. Breathe like this now.' Move the fingers of one hand in a light, rapid rhythm and breathe with her.

Between contractions explain that over the top of each, say, 'wave' or 'mountain', she will breathe like this to let the womb tighten freely and get on with its good work of opening up to let the baby be born. 'These big contractions are doing most work. They are *good* ones, though they may not feel like it at the moment!' Reassure her that you will stay with her and help her, and that you can work together. (Indicate that this is not simply something you are doing *for* her, of which she is the passive recipient, but working *together*.)

Rest a hand on the fundus with the next contraction and, breathing with her as it starts, ask her as the contraction becomes difficult to control, to open her eyes. Interrupt the rhythm only to say Good or give other appropriate praise. Encourage her to give several long blows out at the end of the contraction, and do this with her if she has been breathing very rapidly and lightly for a large part of the contraction. If she is obviously overbreathing, however, do not do this.

Freshen her up with ice or a wash and give more praise and explanations of what is happening between contractions. You are now in a position to gauge the intensity of contractions and hence to estimate approximately whether she is acting appropriately or overreacting. If she is overreacting dramatically she may need to talk things out between contractions and to have an opportunity to express her fears. You might ask 'Have you brothers and sisters? How many are there in your family?' 'Did your mother have a good time when she had her babies? Did she ever talk about it?' 'What did your sister tell you about when she had her baby?' Give accurate information when she has been misled. Give firm guidance and positive assurance that everything is all right. If she can listen to her own baby's heartbeats this may be reassuring; if you have an opportunity to do this indicate with your finger the pulse of the beating heart. After doing this smile at her and if everything is normal *tell* her 'The baby's fine. Everything is just right. You are doing very well.'

Touch is important. It gives comfort, and can communicate to a woman that she is not alone in her ordeal. At the same time it can give a nonverbal message which can be quite specific. Thus it can be used to control the rate and depth of breathing, as well as in stroking the forehead, patting the hand, or lightly stroking the area over the cervix. Where communication in verbal language is limited, touch is of paramount importance. Do not hold a woman's hand, or she may grip it as if it were a life-line. Hold her wrist lightly instead.

After 8 centimetres women frequently lose the rhythm of light, quick breathing at the height of the contraction. If easy breathing is interrupted because of uncontrollable feelings of stress, or because of involuntary breath-holding before she is fully dilated, tell the woman to blow out quickly like 'blowing a balloon away from you', and do this with her. Between the next two contractions explain how she is to blow crisply through pursed lips and then continue to breathe lightly, without pausing.

In cases of severe back pain, massage of the sacrolumbar region can be very helpful. Help the woman to turn over on her side or in the front lateral, with a pillow under the upper flexed leg. Massage firmly with the heel of the palm, moving the flesh on the bone, with a circular movement. Sometimes firm pressure is in itself sufficient. Sometimes a hot-water bottle in the small of the back achieves the same result. A pack used for keeping picnic food hot or cold is ideal for this purpose, and can be reheated in hot water in a hospital wash basin, or used cold, since in cases of acute back pain a cold pack may be useful.* Sit, or stand, facing the mother, so that you can still counsel her, and she can see your face.

As the fetal head descends, back pain may move lower, until she feels an intolerable sensation of distension at the base of the spine and around the anus. Ask her Where do you feel it? If she indicates that this is where the pain is, look pleased and surprised, and say Oh good! Tell her that this is a sign of progress, and move the hand lower; with a rocking movement of the hand from heel of palm to fingers and back again, massage this area, every now and again moving the hand in a circular movement out over the buttocks and the sides of the pelvis.

With all massage ask the mother to relax the part you are touching and to release *towards* your hands. With back massage it may help her to press back very slightly towards your hand.

Between contractions explain to the mother what the uterus is doing, the presentation of the baby and the shape of the birth canal (in a curve like a half-circle, not in a straight line). Some mothers, and particularly those who are anxious, benefit from being told what they are likely to feel *in advance*.

Do not ask Is this your first? or What do you want, a boy or a girl? A dozen sympathetic nurses have probably asked this already. Find out if she is a primipara or multipara from her record chart, and note any other relevant information.

As the first stage advances she will probably tell you again that it is hurting. *Agree* with her that it hurts, and add 'It's very hard work, isn't it? But you are working very well with your breathing.' If she is distressed find out if analgesic or other aid is available. (Sometimes if one is sitting with a patient, staff may think that no other assistance is needed or desirable, and that in some way it would be a 'failure of method' if the woman were given medication. Be careful that you do not give the impression that because you are giving a patient support she is on no account to be offered drugs.)

If a woman starts to shiver during transition a hot-water bottle or heated pack at the feet can help if it is permitted, and firm massage of

* The Trice instant cold pack, produced by Bowaters of Sunbury-on-Thames, England, does not need to be cooled in a refrigerator.

the adductors. Do not pile on more blankets, as the weight can be uncomfortable at this phase of labour. Massage the inner thighs with warm, relaxed hands curved to the shape of the mother's legs, from knee up almost to the perineum lightly and then *firmly* down again, asking her to relax towards your hands and to let the muscles around the baby's head bulge forward and down towards your hands, 'like a heavy hammock' or 'a large bag of curd cheese' or 'a jelly bag', or some other analogy appropriate to the culture. This feeling of release of the pelvic-floor musculature may be difficult to obtain. Once a good personal relationship is achieved in between contractions cup your hand under one of her breasts and gently move it up and down. Ask her to feel the weight of her own loose breast, and tell her it is like this 'down below'—soft and heavy. She can help the birth 'by letting the muscles go limp and very, very heavy like this'. Sometimes the words *sweet* and *good* are also apposite; sweet, particularly, may suggest the release associated with sexual delight, and pleasure in parts of the body which may be culturally linked with dirt, defecation, uncleanliness, sin and shame.

As she enters the second stage urge her to let the baby press down and help the head to bulge forward rather than telling her to push or bear down. Never say More, More or Harder, Harder, as this can result in unnecessary straining and wasted effort. Concentrate instead on regulation of the breathing, correct rounded-back posture, and pelvic-floor release. If she seems fearful tell her she will feel 'very warm down there' as the baby's head presses against the perineum. Reassure her that this is a good feeling and means the baby will soon be born.

If she is flat on a delivery table, a most difficult position in which to bear down smoothly and easily, climb up behind her and support head and shoulders, or stand close with an arm around her. If standing, fix one foot on the rail running along the base of the table (if there is one) for extra support.

Explain what things are for in the delivery room, so allaying anxiety and helping the woman to relate to her surroundings. Introduce doctors and nurses if names are known: 'This is Dr. X. He's going to help you have the baby.'

Keep her head dropped, *not* pressed, forward on her chest for bearing down. If she hollows her back put a hand under, and ask her to press down against your hand.

If you are able to assist delivery with your instructions to the labouring woman—you should be ready to defer to midwife or obstetrician delivering, and you can ascertain this by simply asking 'Do you want me to go on telling her what to do, or would you rather take over here?'—conduct the second stage with slow, measured breathing to meet contractions, two, three or four sustained held breaths for bearing down, and slow breaths at the end of each contraction. Encourage the mother to rest completely between. Do not direct the woman to hold on to each breath with such desperation that she becomes exhausted. Avoid shouting or peremptory commands.

If the perineum seems unduly stretched get her to 'blow away' several contractions, breathing with her. Since you will have a mask on by now, be careful that your speech is distinct and that you use gesture to supplement verbal instructions. Do not forget that your eyes can betray your feelings, and can either look anxious or smiling.

Once the occiput is clearly visible and about the size of the rim of a small coffee cup, tell her, and show her with a mirror if she is happy to look. Tell her that she needs to open her eyes both so that you can work together very carefully and so that she can see her baby at once. Meet the next contractions with slow breathing as before, but then, as the urge increases, change to quick breathing. She holds her breath only when this is inevitable and compelling, that is 'holding your breath when you must', breathing again rapidly as soon as comfortable. In this way the head will ease out more gently.

As the head crowns get her to pant slowly. Explain the function of the mucus catheter: 'They always clean out the breathing passages like this.' Encourage and help her by propping her up to watch the birth, and if attendants seem unaware of the desirability of this, ask if she may hold the baby immediately, unwashed and naked. If she wishes, and if doctor agrees, help her to put the baby to the breast immediately, before the separation and delivery of the placenta. This will help the uterus to contract strongly.

Should the child need resuscitation, tell her calmly that 'many babies need to be helped to breathe. We may have to wait ten minutes.' Never tell a mother her baby is perfectly all right if it is not. If the child is obviously not responding to life and she asks about it, say 'The doctors are working with the baby'. Then, later, with further questions, one can add, 'They are working very hard. They are doing all they can.' In this way, with the slow passage of time, the woman has the chance to adjust gradually to the idea of loss, should the baby not live. This is very much better than the dishonesty which stems from the attendant's own fear of the emotions of grief which are aroused.

Let the mother handle the baby, explore its body, examine its limbs, fingers and toes and cuddle it. If she needs suturing, this may be best done whilst the baby is in her arms, and the whole anti-climax then becomes much more tolerable. Tell her she has done well. If there is any doubt in her mind about her performance, reassure her that she has been splendid, that all has gone very well, that she has a lovely baby and that she is a good mother.

18

The Stress Phase of Labour

There is one period of labour which some of us tend to skip over lightly, or to feel that there is little we can do to help with, except to rely on medication and support given at the time. This is the period right at the end of the first stage, lasting from perhaps half an hour to three hours, when stress is probably greater for the woman than it is at any other time during the childbirth. This is conveniently labelled *transition*, because it is a sign of progress towards the expulsive stage, and is a bridge between the first and second stages of labour.

There are really two rather different subjective phenomena in labour, both of which may be labelled *transition* and which may also overlap.

One is the *storm at sea* . It is the time right at the end of the first stage, when contractions are tumultuous, powerful, more or less unpredictable, and possibly arrythmic. The labouring woman may become confused, irritable, despairing, or, if given inadequate support or deprived of the feeling of personal identity by conveyer-belt hospital routines, panic-stricken and distressed. She may start to shake, feel very chilled, and vomit. Low backache, especially in the case of posterior presentations of the vertex, may be intense and worry her more than the sensations from contractions. She also tends to lose her bearings, in time, spatial geography and her environment generally, and faces stresses perhaps not dissimilar to those of an astronaut without companions, completely alone in space.

It is because of this disorientation that techniques of stimulating the attention are particularly appropriate at this phase. Those stimuli include:

signals by *touch*, including massage; signals which say, in effect, 'I am here with you and helping you. I am sharing the experience in some measure.'

encouraging *words* and praise, which convey the message 'Everything is all right. You're doing fine. You need have no doubts about your ability to do this.'

refreshing with ice water or ice chips, sucked or applied to the skin; with fresh air or a cool fan or change of posture; or change of surroundings.

prompting to open the *eyes* and avoid descending into the long, dark tunnel of private nightmare during contractions; being able to say, in effect, 'We are in this together'. This involves eye movement, and signals for attention emanating from the eyes.

As her labour sweeps forward the woman is propelled out into a bizarre world of subjective experience, one which, for the primipara, is amazingly and utteringly new, but which for each woman in each labour brings surprises and sensations she has not experienced before. Her body is like a craft which is forcing her forward into this intense experience; it is no longer the body with which she was familiar and which she thought she knew, but one capable of immense power and energy. This force emanating involuntarily from her body outstrips intellect or exercises or any of the carefully rehearsed techniques. She may feel that it is the creative force of life finding expression through her body. For many women this can be a terrifying and alarming, or magnificent and intensely awe-inspiring, experience.

The antenatal teacher sets the scene for this experience by her own attitudes. In a way we have written the overture to what is to follow, and have, by our personal feelings about labour, created the mood for a woman's own experience of birth.

Sometimes she has deliberately avoided describing the tumult and thunder of physical forces and emotions often involved in transition. She may have understated the case, perhaps because she is not very confident about her capacity to handle this experience herself.

Or perhaps she has boldly oversimplified, and presented it all in terms of sheer pain. In both cases it seems to me that teachers are not giving their pupils all that they might. We must remember that the sensations experienced during transition are all *signs of progress*, and that the labouring woman can be taught to recognize them gladly. They then become reassuring rather than alarming.

The other phenomenon commonly associated with transition is the *catch in the throat*. It may occur at any time during this phase, and with or without the other subjective phenomena. This is the beginning of the expulsive reflex, often experienced initially as an involuntarily held breath. This heralds the second stage.

Antenatal teachers are inclined to view this spontaneous urge with deep suspicion, and to warn all pupils that they must on no account allow themselves to push until they have been examined *per vaginam* and instructed to push by the midwife or doctor. They may even tell their pupils that to bear down before instructed will lacerate the cervix and cause the fetal head to be 'hammered' against it. To cope with the urge various extremely useful techniques are taught which allow the diaphragm to be lifted off the fundus, so avoiding the piston-like movement which we term *bearing down*. There are several things we should keep in mind however:

Firstly, the woman may be able to control her own voluntary bearing down for some time, but the uterus will continue to contract and to work to expel its contents. No amount of breathing techniques can prevent this. If the uterus is contracting hard, the woman can blow till she is blue in the face, but the presenting part will still be pressed down through the cervix. She has in no way failed, nor is she doing her exercises incorrectly, if this happens. It is simply that her uterus works that way.

Secondly, doctors and midwives are not always available or willing to examine vaginally at the end of the first stage, and particularly if the patient is resting and seems not far advanced in labour. There is a tendency to examine vaginally as little as possible because of the risk of infection, and some obstetricians argue, sensibly, that the woman will have to push anyway when she is really ready. In this it is the antenatal teachers who seem to be demanding techniques which do not accord with Nature and the obstetricians and midwives who often believe in letting Nature take its course. It would be a pity if we so trained women that they were left desperately blowing and trying not to push when the baby was ready to be pressed down the birth canal, and when active cooperation with uterine activity could bring them enormous satisfaction and a sense of well-being. (The baby, of course, will be born anyway.)

Thirdly, by stating that the woman must not push at all until given permission to do so, we may imply that from that point on she must exert all her power to expel the baby, without consideration of the strength or inner pattern of each contraction, or of the state of the perineum. Having been taught by our classes that her body is not to be trusted in transition, she then approaches the second stage with the same sense of mistrust, and tackles contractions mechanically, without the subtlety and finesse which comes from the ability to 'listen to' her body and to follow the instructions of her uterus—rather like an orchestra following the conductor.

With this in mind it could be pointed out to pupils that the first time they get a catch in the throat of course they may find themselves bearing down a bit. That is natural. They will know that with the next contraction, or perhaps the one after that, when the same feeling comes, they can blow out (or whatever other technique they have been taught).

The blowing breathing for this phase is either *candle breathing* or *blowing the balloon away* (see page 190). The pattern varies with the expulsive urge. As the urge comes it can be handled by 'blowing the candle flame out'. If the woman overreacts and tends to blow so hard that there is an almost complete gaseous exchange, it is better to ask her to imagine blowing a balloon. If at any time the desire to push becomes too strong to be dealt with in this way, she should be reassured that it is all right to push. There is no reason to be anxious, and certainly no reason for us to suggest to our pupils that if they surrender happily to this urge they will be 'torn to ribbons'! From that point it is a natural development of method for the woman to learn how to 'blow away' a second-stage contraction when the advancing fetal head is causing stress to perineal tissues.

Sometimes the expulsive urge never establishes itself very strongly, and everyone, including the labouring woman, is wondering whether it is all right to bear down. On examination the vagina and cervix are found to be one canal, but the woman is still happily managing to breathe her way through contractions and does not feel any urge to push. In either of these cases suggest that with the next contraction the woman starts with slow breathing, as she will have been doing before, but as the contraction builds up she takes a complete breath and holds on to it; if she is ready to push this is then followed by a feeling, however slight and indefinable, of bearing down as intra-abdominal pressure builds up. With each ensuing contraction the feeling will increase, until she finds she is well into the swing of the second stage. If, however, and in the absence of vaginal examination, she takes a breath like this and holds it, and it is followed by pain, this is an indication that she is not yet ready for pushing, and she should go back to former breathing for transition.

Any description of the sensations of the expulsive reflex should take into account the fact that, even though extremely strong, it brings with it a satisfying feeling of physical efficiency, and sensations, resulting from the downward pressure of the fetal head, which lead to an 'opening up' feeling in the vagina which can also be highly pleasurable. At first, before the fetus has made its journey round the arc of the birth canal, it may feel as if the baby is emerging through the anus. This can be an alarming sensation. But gradually it becomes clear that the baby's head is bulging farther forward. It is rather a surge of passionate urgency comparable only to the mounting desire with which a woman approaches orgasm in happy love-making.

If a labour is flowing well, there is everything to be gained from the woman keeping consciously in tune with her contractions, and remaining aware of and cooperating with the physiological process, and she can be given emotional support to handle her contractions without the need for drugs. Her own wishes regarding pharmacological pain relief should always be respected in this, and the choice be hers, not the attendants. Given instruction beforehand and support at the time, she need not feel that she has in any way failed if she requires pain relief in the latter part of the first stage. She can still assist actively with the second stage and work with her midwife to give birth to her baby in joy.

The Second Stage

Now the living child
Long cherished by the mother beneath her heart,
Fills the gateway of life.
There is room to pass safely through.
The child slips downward,
It becomes visible,
It bursts forth into the light of day.

Polynesian*

The second stage of labour is usually considered a time when athletic effort is necessary. It is commonly a matter of straining and pushing to force the baby down through the birth canal, a process during which women go red in the face, when their neck muscles stand out rigid and hard, and when they puff and grunt with their desperate attempt to push the head down just a little lower so that they receive the praise and approval which seems so slow in coming from their attendants. Push! Push! Again! commands the obstetrician. Hold it. Go on. Harder! Harder! Push . . . push, push . . . push . . . push . . . again . . . again . . . again. Come on, you can do it harder than that! Sweat drips off the woman as she strains harder, teeth clenched, facial muscles taut, brow furrowed with effort, fists clenched as she pulls on her arms. Little blood vessels burst in her eyes and face, and all too often she looks as if a whirlwind had swept over her by the

* Quoted in David Melzer's *Birth* (New York, Ballantine Books, 1973).

time she is delivered, and has scarlet blotches, aching neck, and even a sore throat the day after.

No one would think that there is a uterus in there doing the work, and, in most cases, working perfectly efficiently to get the baby born. No one would think that Nature had devised a system of physiological machinery which causes the baby to be gently but firmly pressed down the birth canal into the outside world.

For whatever 'reason' a hurried delivery is done, although it involves more haste, it almost invariably means less speed. For the woman quickly becomes exhausted and confused with straining, and loses her ability for complete and precise neuromuscular awareness and control. And not only this; she forfeits the capacity for acute sensitivity, particularly of the area around the birth canal itself and on the perineum, so that she is incapable of the delicate adjustment necessary to allow the baby to ooze out slowly and gently, rather than to be propelled like a cork out of a champagne bottle. In losing this capacity, she also loses the pleasurable sensations of warmth around the vagina which come with the slow descent of the baby's head, a relaxed pelvic floor and perineum, and the accompanying feelings of opening up as if a flower were opening wide all its petals.

A typical description of the second stage from the stand-point of the textbook on obstetrics says that

she must 'force down' and contract her abdominal muscles, while bracing herself against a solid object. She pulls on the handbars, and at the same time bears down as hard, and for as long a period, as she can. With each contraction the pressure on the perineum and rectum stimulates the patient to move towards the head of the table and out of the best position. Shoulder braces will prevent this. . . . At the stage where the head is passing through the introitus the patient has the sensation of being torn apart.*

Let us examine more closely exactly what is happening when a woman is encouraged to bear down in this way:

She is told that she is bearing down with her abdominal muscles, whereas in fact she does not need actively to contract abdominal musculature to push. All that is necessary is that she *stabilizes* her

* Harry Oxorn and William R. Foote, *Human Labor and Birth* (London, Butterworths, 1968).

lateral abdominal muscles as she holds her breath. She then *releases* the main bulge of the abdominal wall, so that the lower abdomen is pressed out and forward as the bearing down movement passes through the birth canal to fan out the tissues of the vagina. If she is struggling to pull in the abdominal wall she is wasting energy.

Note that she is also instructed to pull on hand grips, which entails contraction of muscles in the arms, shoulders and neck. This is another way to waste energy, and is almost invariably associated with heavy, gasping breathing and the risks of hyperventilation. The tendency will be for her also to throw her head back, lifting her chin up from her chest, and to bear down using her throat muscles. The result may be a noisy second stage and aching throat and shoulders after the baby is born.

This mother is described as struggling away from the sensations on the perineum, with a result that she moves towards the head of the delivery table, and the remedy proposed is to prevent her doing this with shoulder restrainers. She moves in this direction largely because she is told to pull with her arms, and a more humane remedy for her movement up the delivery table would be to tell her to relax her arms by her side, and to prop her up well with four or five pillows or a firm foam wedge. If the husband is helping a pillow can be placed in the crook of his elbow too, and he then supports her shoulders and neck with the firm base provided by his arm and the pillow together.

She is told to bear down as hard as she can for as long as she can, without regard to the different kinds of contraction which occur in the second stage, to the position of the baby's head, or the stresses on the perineum as the head crowns. Not all second-stage contractions are alike; some are powerful, others gentle, and the woman who has been taught to trust and work with her body, instead of fighting and denying it, can respond appropriately to the different contractions if given emotional support to do so. Moreover if she bears down forcefully and without finesse once the head is on the perineum she is in danger of subjecting the perineal tissues to unnecessary stress. This is where cooperation with her midwife or obstetrician is all important, and where instruction to breathe out the baby's head, interspersed with pushing, can be very helpful.

Where there is a flexible approach to the second stage, women can cooperate harmoniously not only with their attendants but with the contracting uterus. As a result they are in tune with second-stage contractions to a degree that is remarkable to anyone who has never seen the way in which women can achieve complete, unstrained neuromuscular coordination for expulsion.

Women frequently become insensitive to the rhythm of uterine contractions in the second stage because they are struggling to obey their attendants and to put their all into each push. Unfortunately they are not usually encouraged to 'listen' to the contractions. Both the amount of effort required by each contraction and the timing of that effort is dictated by the uterus itself. Rarely is any contraction 'all push'. Instead the urge to bear down comes in different waves with each contraction, sometimes missing a contraction altogether. These waves are like surges, sweeping through each contraction between two and four times. They can be compared with the surges of desire which occur in coitus once the woman has attained the orgasmic platform preceding climax, that is, these pushing surges are *clustered*.

If she is anxiously straining to bear down all the time, regardless of the waves of desire to push, she may miss the surges altogether, and with them the satisfying sense of psychophysical coordination and *sexual* activity which can accompany normal, unforced bearing down. Indeed, she can be working so hard, and may have started doing so even before the natural urge was there, that she never really wants to push, but only does so because she is told to.

The urge to push can be intensely passionate and overwhelming or much more muted. In each case it is a satisfying activity bringing with it fulfilment and peace as each contraction fades away. The woman who tends to be inhibited should be encouraged to respond wholeheartedly and with no holding back to whatever she feels, and be praised for her response. ('You did that beautifully. Just go with it. That's right. Let it flow right through.') She should never be told to push, or commanded to 'hang on to it' or to 'push in to your back passage'.

For a large part of the second stage in a great many labours, and particularly primiparous deliveries, the woman *wants* to push, and to throw herself into the activity of bearing down with all her might, and can take an almost reckless joy in the action of the second stage. The stimulus is there, and she has intense pleasure in responding to it. But this is spontaneous response to an inbuilt stimulus—one that needs no commands from outside, no cheerleading from attendants. The instructions are coming in no uncertain terms from inside her, from her own contracting uterus, and she can respond to them. The task of doctors and nurses is to give emotional support and to create an atmosphere in which a woman can confidently listen to her uterus and adapt herself to its rhythm, in this way.

There are women who panic in the second stage and who resist urges which are evidently there, for some reason or other fight their bodies as they are involved in the processes of expulsion, contract muscles involuntarily, and who cannot face the idea of pushing the baby out. A woman caught in this fearful conflict with her own body is quite different from that of the woman who simply 'does not want to push yet' or 'not with this one', or who wants to push 'but only gently'.

It is rarely sheer pain as such that creates this conflict. Usually the woman is fearful that to push would injure her or the baby. Sometimes these fears can be dispelled by accurate, precise information which helps her to understand that the lining of the birth canal is composed of soft, stretchable tissues which can open up like a fan with the pressure of the baby's head against them. She may need to be told that it is safer for a baby to be born vaginally, even though the birth canal seems surprisingly constricting and the processes of birth very hard on the baby, than through an abdominal incision. She may need explanation about moulding of the fetal head, of how it is rather like a large grapefruit as it is pressed down the arc of the birth canal, and of how the parietal bones can move towards each other, and even overlap slightly at the line of the suture between them and at the anterior and posterior fontanelles.

Other women resist by involuntary contraction of muscles in the pelvic floor at the base of the spine and in the buttocks because they fear that they are going to 'make a mess', and associate the sensations of rectal pressure with all the social taboos on defecation in public or in unsuitable places. The woman who is fearful that the baby is 'coming out of the wrong hole' or that she really needs a bedpan, rather than being instructed to push without discretion, should be reminded to 'open up below', be 'soft and loose', and 'help the baby's head bulge forward'.

Some women simply do not get an urge to bear down. Very often this occurs when the mother is lying flat, and if she is helped into a squatting or kneeling position, and remains so for a few contractions, the urge comes. It is only in modern hospitals that a supine position is considered suitable for the second stage and in which the woman is expected either to lie flat or to be spread-eagled in lithotomy like a beetle on its back. In other cultures the labouring woman squats, sits or kneels supported by helpers, letting gravity help fetal descent and rotation. But even when a physiologically correct position for bearing down is adopted, some women get but slight desire to push. Sometimes, as I have already indicated, this is because it is too soon. Sometimes it is because instructions are given which do not correspond to the height of the bearing down reflexes occurring in wave-like clusters with each contraction once the second stage is well established, and, as we have seen, varying in duration and intensity with contraction.

There are other women, experiencing a precipitate second stage, and in particular multigravidae, who do not need to bear down actively because the uterus is doing the work for them, who get no urge to push for most of the second stage, and for whom forceful pushing would mean putting unnecessary strain on the perineum.

Because the urge to push comes in waves of bearing down surges, the deeply held breath at the onset of a contraction, terminated only by a gasping explosion of air as she can hold on no longer, and followed again by another great inhalation is entirely inappropriate for the second stage. It is bound to result in tension. It is also very doubtful whether breathing like this allows a woman to fill her lungs to the best advantage. Certainly divers are instructed to avoid taking one deep breath and trying to hold on to it under water, and are taught instead to do a series of quick breaths, and then hold on to the last one as they dive under, in order to get the maximum amount of air in the lungs.

If one watches a mammal giving birth a very different pattern of breathing in the expulsive stage is observed. A cat or dog breathes rapidly, holds the breath, and then breathes rapidly again, holds the breath and so on, till the end of the contraction. When an orang-outang in Dresden Zoo delivered I was fortunate to be there within a few hours of the birth and was able to closely question the zoo attendant who had witnessed the birth.

The male orang had kept the female on the move throughout the first stage, nipping her from behind so that she did not settle down. In the second stage she crouched, her upper torso bent forward, breathing quickly, and every now and again holding her breath. (I checked this with the attendant, and myself enacted the second stage as he described it, and he was enthusiastic in his approval of my performance of an orang-outang about to deliver.) Incidentally, once the head was on the perineum the male orang applied his lips to the occiput of the baby's head, which because he has both an inner and an outer lip, created a vacuum similar to the rubber lip on a Thermos flask, and delivered the baby by vacuum extraction.

The sheep breathes in a similar way, and I acquired the confidence to breathe in this way when giving birth to my own twins, after having watched a sheep delivering a few hours before I went into labour. Consequently it has become known to my students as the *sheep breathing*.

In the second stage the woman meets her contraction with slow, steady breathing, meanwhile concentrating on the wave of the contraction, and waiting for it to build up. As it becomes more powerful and impelling, she moves up to quicker, shallower breathing, until she is doing mouth-centred breathing. The surge of desire to bear down comes towards her, and she automatically finds herself breathing rather more deeply, with more pronounced, but not heavy, rapid breathing. This is almost invariably accompanied by changes in facial expression which are those of sexual excitement, and with which the husband is usually happily familiar. Her face is pinker, her eyes shining, hair damp.

Suddenly her breath is held involuntarily as the urge to bear down becomes overpowering. She holds her breath at this point, her lips parted, jaw relaxed as she continues to hold her breath, head inclined forward on her chest, arms and shoulders relaxed, 'leaning' on the contraction as she does so, and allowing the bearing-down movement to pass down through the uterus until the vagina opens up. She concentrates on the sensation of pelvic-floor release and relaxation towards the area of greatest pressure, distension and heat, which she will already have learned with Touch Relaxation, thus working with the contraction to 'open the door' for her baby to be born. As soon as the surge recedes she returns to mouth-centred breathing, waiting for the next surge, holds her breath again when the urge reaches its peak, and so on. In this way she can bear down without straining two to four times with each contraction, and as the contraction dies away, her breathing slows down and becomes rather deeper, terminating in a long, slow 'resting breath' similar to that at the end of first-stage contractions, as she sinks back to rest completely between contractions.

In all this it is not a matter of a certain required number of deep breaths which have to be taken in and held. If we teach women *how* to push and how to breathe for expulsion we must make it clear that we have given them the basic tools, the instruments they can use, but that the manner in which they use them is a matter for decision at the time, a decision which is only partly rational and intellectual, and largely quite spontaneous.

The well-prepared woman often remarks, 'It seemed quite natural' . . . 'I don't know how I could have done anything else'. This is what techniques are for, whether they are techniques of sex play, breastfeeding, child-rearing, or for use in labour. They are only perfectly used when they are no longer obvious, and when they take their place in a harmonious flow of activity which seems inevitable and natural.

A woman in the second stage does not need to press her lips together or grit her teeth in order to bear down. Instead there is a slight smile, and the parted lips are soft as the unfolding and opening vaginal lips. If she has practised pelvic-floor release with this association in mind beforehand she can consciously use the idea of a relaxed mouth to achieve good perineal release.

The position in which a woman bears down with greatest ease is that in which her back is rounded, and her knees bent and drawn up. Some women like this position on the side, and then they assume the traditional left lateral English position for expulsion, still favoured by some midwives. This is a position which may be the most comfortable for the mother when the baby is in a posterior position, and has still not rotated at the onset of the expulsive stage. It allows the mother to have firm back support from her husband's hand, permits the midwife to control the delivery of the head, and also favours rotation of the head if she lies on the side opposite to that on which the baby's back is lying.

Probably most women like the dorsal position, however, and this is the one preferred by obstetricians and many midwives. The back should be well and firmly supported, with the trunk raised at whatever angle is most comfortable *for the mother*. Some women suffer from postural hypotension and feel giddy if they lie low, and they are best sitting up, with the base of the spine resting flat on the delivery table or bed. The back should be a convex curve whether the woman is lying, sitting, squatting, crouching or kneeling, all of which are good alternatives, provided that whoever is delivering feels they can cope with these positions. There is an obvious advantage in being able to really bear *down*, and letting gravity help the descent of the baby. The legs should be relaxed, knees and ankles rotated outwards to avoid bearing down 'through the legs' with consequent cramp. Arms should also be flexed and relaxed. The woman's head should be dropped forward on the chest to aid bearing down and to avoid straining with the throat muscles.

Labour chairs, or beds based on the idea of the medieval labour stool or the commode are being used experimentally in the United States and Scandinavian countries. A recent development in Britain is a delivery chair designed by Renou with assistance from myself, which is similar in design to a patio chair with inclined back rest, elbow supports which adjust to suit the woman, and adjustable foot rests. A 'bean bag' of polystyrene foam granules can also be a comfortable and easily adapted back support.

For the obstetrician who is accustomed to doing routine episiotomies, and who feels that delivery without episiotomy runs unnecessary risks for both mother and baby, the unforced second stage may provide an alternative. He is probably used to seeing women bearing down with all that lies in their power, being encouraged to do so by a team of nurses and doctors who are so caught up in the action that they are often bearing down themselves too[1] This enforced activity starts at the moment when the woman is pronounced fully dilated and proceeds at a rapid pace until the baby is delivered. Such a woman requires an episiotomy to avoid not only superficial perineal laceration, but button-hole tears in the mucosa of the vagina.

Any decision to act conservatively and see whether episiotomy is required with that particular delivery must be accompanied by a method of conducting the second stage so that the final descent of the fetal presenting part on to the perineum, the stretching of tissues, and the delivery of the baby, take place slowly, gently, and with delicate precision. To do this full cooperation is necessary between the woman and her attendants, and even before the crowning occurs —often well before this point is reached—the woman is asked to 'blow contractions away'. (This she will have learned to do anyway for coping with transition.) When the uterus alone is permitted to get on with its work of pressing the baby through the birth canal, without any extra expulsive effort coming from the mother, and when with light blowing breaths she stops herself from bearing down, the delivery can be much better controlled.

Sometimes women seem to get disoriented at this phase of labour —not because of fear or pain but because their bodies feel no longer like the bodies with which they are familiar, and they find it difficult to coordinate in such a way that they are relaxed or know what they are doing with the pelvic-floor musculature. It can feel as if the top half of one's body has become detached from the lower half. There are two ways in which support can be given at this phase:

The labouring woman can be provided with a mirror-view of the dilating vagina, so that visually the perineum and birth canal are once again conceptually incorporated into her body percept—the importance of which is already discussed in Chapter 8. Many women who have been to classes like to use a delivery mirror, which the husband holds slanted above his wife's abdomen, or, with the midwife's permission, above her thighs. But if a woman is well propped up she can often herself see from the crowning on. I think it helps many women to see what is happening as they breathe and push and breathe again once the head is on the perineum, and that this gives meaning to sensations which otherwise can be confusing, disturbing and frequently alarming. If that is the top of the baby's head, no wonder she feels these strange pricking sensations of stretching as her body opens wide.

The birth canal can feel very little like that part of the body with which one so carefully did pelvic floor exercises during pregnancy. For this reason there is little point in anyone saying to the woman about to deliver: Relax your pelvic floor. If, however, she is asked to relax her *mouth*, letting her lips part and soften, with her throat and neck released, and her cheeks plumped up in a smile—an action she can rehearse beforehand in classes—the pelvic-floor musculature will offer minimal resistance, and there is a resulting increased flexibility of perineal tissues.

So these two things, relaxation of the mouth and throat, and use of a delivery mirror, can together increase the woman's conscious joyful and controlled participation in the act of birth. They can allow the head to be delivered over two or three contractions, the shoulders to slide out after a pause, either with or between contractions, and then the rest of the body to slither out and into the outstretched arms of an eager, laughing mother, who, far from being exhausted, is immediately ready to take on the tasks of motherhood.

Such an approach to the controlled and gentle management of the second stage needs, of necessity, to be a team process, and involves everyone working with the labouring woman, her antenatal teachers, whoever is giving support and companionship in labour, and those delivering her.

Curtain Up on Parenthood

20

Talking about the Newborn Baby

The ideal context in which to discuss with prospective parents the appearance and behaviour of the new baby is the group to which new parents return, bringing with them their own babies, as soon as possible after delivery. It is often arranged in classes as the occasion for a labour report, so that class members can hear what happened in labour and how the woman coped. But this other function, of giving expectant parents an opportunity to see, handle and talk about the baby, is also very important, and should not be overlooked in the emphasis on labour.

The First Breath

Discussion usually crops up spontaneously about how a baby breathes, and why, and what happens when things go wrong, especially in classes in which husbands are participating. The ante-natal teacher should be able to describe vividly in simple terms the enormous circulatory changes that take place at delivery, and the things that can be done to help when the baby does not breathe easily.

It sounds simple to say 'the baby breathes', but in the short space of a few minutes enormous changes take place, and the child adjusts from a being in which food is oxygenated outside its own body to a complete individual with lungs oxygenating its blood. Let us first see again what happens to the baby inside the uterus, looking especially at the way in which the circulation of the blood takes place. At the end of pregnancy all major nerve pathways of the baby's central nervous system are almost completely formed, but they are like a telephone exchange with few incoming calls, and with not so very many going out either. There is also an intricate plumbing system of heart and blood vessels already fully developed.

After birth the two sides of the heart are completely separate, each with a collecting chamber—the atrium—and a pumping chamber—the ventricle. The right heart collects the blood streaming in from all parts of the body along the great veins and pumps it to the lungs. The left heart collects blood from the lungs and pumps it through the aorta to all the arteries of the body after birth.

The lungs are like a sponge. All the blood flowing to the lungs from the right heart passes through tiny vessels in the thin partition walls between the air holes in the sponge. In this way the lungs provide a huge area for the exchange of oxygen and carbon dioxide between the blood and the air which has been breathed into the cells. The air is changed by movement of the chest wall, as if you alternately squeezed and let go the sponge in a bowl of water. But *before birth* it is squeezed up tightly and the air cells are empty, or contain only a thin film of the amniotic fluid in which the baby is floating.

The placenta is even more like a sponge than the lungs. It grew from the egg cell as part of the fetus, not the mother, and by the time it is fully developed, at about three-months' gestation, it is a large thick plaque attached to the baby by the umbilical cord. Its roots are attached to the inside wall of the uterus, like a cushion of moss inside a hollow tree stump.

The baby's blood from the left heart comes down two arteries in the umbilical cord, flows through the walls of the cells of the spongy placenta and then back to the baby through the cord by a single umbilical vein, joining up with the main veins in the abdomen to flow back to the right heart. So, just as for air in the lungs, there is a large area of contact where the mother's circulating blood is separated from the baby's circulating blood by only a paper-thin wall. This allows not only oxygen and carbon dioxide but also simple food molecules from the mother's blood, and waste products from the baby's blood, to diffuse across, as if through a very fine sieve.

Before birth the baby has no need of blood passing through its lungs. The circulation develops two routes by which blood from the right heart can by-pass the lungs, go straight to the left heart, and from there round the baby's body. First, there is a hole left in the partition between the two collecting chambers of the right and left heart. The sides of the hole overlap, like a flap valve. This is called the *foramen ovale*. Blood from the main vein of the lower half of the body is directed straight through the hole to the left heart, to travel from there to all the baby's tissues. Second, there is an artery which connects the main vessel from the right heart to the lungs to the main artery which leads from the left heart to the rest of the body. It is called the *ductus arteriosus*. This is short and thick, and also directly by-passes the lungs, but the amount of blood that flows through it depends on the pressure difference between its two ends.

The blood pressure which the heart develops depends on the resistance to flow in the tissues through which the blood is passing. This is controlled largely by the tone of the muscles in the artery walls, and this, in turn, by nerve signals from the brain. This is the way in which blood supply to different parts of the body is regulated according to their needs at different times. Before birth there are few signals from the brain; all the arteries are relaxed and flow is easy. So the pressure in the left heart is low. The lungs, as we have seen, are squeezed up, with a restricted blood flow through them. The pressure in the right heart is relatively high—slightly higher than that in the left heart.

It has been demonstrated from work on lambs that the baby makes respiratory movements in utero. Simple reflex movements of, for example, the head, start very early on in pregnancy, and gradually movement is extended to other groups of muscles, including those involved in respiration. The baby thus rehearses respiration long before it actually needs to breathe.

The teacher might ask the class: 'Why do you think a newborn baby breathes?' There are two enormous changes for the baby when it emerges from the uterus. First, the strong contractions of the uterine wall cut off the maternal blood supply to the placenta. Second, the placenta starts to separate from the uterus. Oxygen can no longer diffuse through to the baby's blood in the same quantity and gradually runs short. The first stage of *anoxia* (oxygen lack) is a powerful stimulus to a special part of the brain, and signals begin to pour into it. Then the baby comes out into the world, and with the moment of birth all the sensory nerves are automatically stimulated —sight, sound and touch. Added to these come internal messages from the baby's own muscles and joints as it is suddenly free to move unhindered by the confining walls of the uterus and the birth canal for the very first time. These signals all pour up to the 'gasping centre' of the brain, to trigger off a new wave of outward motor impulses, which themselves trigger off all sorts of activity.

If the newborn baby is put down on a table or bed, it moves its arms, legs, body, and eyes, and probably cries. But if it is wrapped up securely in a warm, quiet shaded place or cuddled peacefully in the mother's arms—so reducing stimuli—it will go to sleep until some internal stimulus, like hunger or a full bowel, or an external stimulus, like loud noise (as from other babies crying in a hospital nursery) wakes it up again.

The first effect of this burst of motor activity in the brain of the newborn baby is on the circulation. The muscle walls of the arteries in the cord contract powerfully and shut down all flow of the baby's blood to the placenta. Blood goes on flowing from the placenta through the cord vein to the baby, however, until most of it is drained and the cord goes white. Often the obstetrician or midwife waits with a hand on the cord until it stops pulsating, and only then clamps it in two places and cuts it between the clamps. This extra blood provides the baby with a greater store of iron for the first three months. If the mother wishes the baby to be delivered on to her abdomen, the cord may be cut earlier to guard against the slight risk of blood draining down into the placenta again.

This is followed by other spectacular changes. The ductus arteriosus contracts down, and finally closes altogether, directing more blood through the lungs. Arteries throughout the body tighten up, and oxygen lack makes them tighten still further. This makes the pressure in the left heart rise above that in the right heart, and the flap valve between the two collecting chambers closes. Now all the blood in the right heart passes through the lungs.

Meanwhile motor signals from the brain are being picked up by all the muscles of the body. The muscles of the chest wall and diaphragm (the great muscle which separates the abdomen from the chest and which thins out and spreads on breathing in, rather like an upside-down umbrella being opened up, so pressing the ribs out) contract strongly. The ribs swing out, the chest expands, and air flows in through the baby's mouth and nose to enter the lungs for the first time. As the lungs expand the pathway for the blood through them also becomes easier.

When the newborn baby takes its first gasp of air, the expiratory centre of the brain is stimulated and the air is squeezed out of the lungs in an active process. The vocal chords too, often share in this burst of activity; they tighten up and the first breath becomes a cry. This does not mean that the baby is unhappy. Later inspiration becomes an active expansion, while breathing out is passive, like a balloon slowly going down.

There are various reasons why a baby may not take a breath in as it is born. Sometimes too few signals are being directed to the brain and the baby is unusually drowsy, perhaps because of drugs that have passed through the mother's bloodstream. Sometimes the air cannot get into the lungs because, for instance, the nose and throat are blocked by mucus. A strong, active baby will manage to get some air in anyway, and squeeze it out again, clearing the passages a bit as it does this, and gradually getting rid of the mucus. It can be helped to do this by lying it down with the head lower than the buttocks so that any mucus present in the air ways begins to drain out. A weak baby, who is already short of oxygen or whose respiratory centre is dulled by anaesthesia, may not be able to get any air into its lungs. There is no expansion to trigger off the expiratory effort which should follow. As oxygen runs short so the brain activity begins to slow down.

Luckily the heart is much less sensitive to oxygen lack than the brain is, and will go on beating at this stage. The first thing is to clear the air passages of nose and throat with gentle suction, either by mouth through a fine tube (a mucus catheter) or with a special controlled suction pump, and this is usually done (often when the baby does not need it), to ensure that the air ways are clear. This may be enough to start breathing, or a few squeezes by hand on the baby's chest, or mouth to mouth breathing may do so. The baby turns pink, its circulatory tone improves and the brain begins to work again.

Soon it starts to breathe for itself and the tube can be taken out. The baby who took some time to breathe may be put in an incubator, where it can be assured of warm, moist air, protection from infection—and constant observation. The incubator provides its own small world for the baby, with perspex walls and with all the conditions of temperature, humidity and gas mixture carefully controlled. Enriching the air the baby breathes at this stage with oxygen up to about 40 per cent is often helpful. But too much oxygen for more than a few days may be harmful. A degenerative condition of the eyes, which can lead to blindness, called *retrolental fibroplasia*, can occur if a baby is kept in 100 per cent oxygen for prolonged periods; another condition of the lungs of premature babies—hyalin membrane disease—is also thought to be connected with high oxygen tensions.

Sometimes cot nursing, with as little moving or touching as possible, is used for shocked babies who have endured a difficult birth, and this extra rest is one of the reasons why mothers may not be allowed to cuddle their babies in the twenty-four hours or so after birth. However, the trend in modern paediatrics is now towards a greater emphasis on the reciprocal needs of mother and baby and on the fostering of the closeness of the mother–child relationship.

The teacher should explain that most babies make these adjustments to life within a matter of seconds after birth. As soon as the chest is free from pressure, even before the rest of the body slides out, a vigorous baby may breathe. In fact a healthy full-term infant will often almost swim out of its mother's body, making strong creeping movements, without further assistance.

As the head first appears it may be blue or purple, and only when the child has taken its first great gasp is it that the skin flushes a bright red as oxygen is carried by the bloodstream through its body. Later on the skin colour settles down to a proper new baby colour, but the baby just a few minutes old often looks lobster-scarlet.

What the Baby Looks Like and What He or She Can Do

The healthy baby's wail is loud and fierce and the muscle tone and colour good. The newborn's condition is estimated according to the Apgar scale, and each child can be given from 1 to 10 points on this scale relating to the degree of vitality it demonstrates, most babies being somewhere between 7 and 10. The baby weighs anything from about 2.5 kg (5.8 lbs) to 4.5 kg (10 lbs) and is 43 cm (17 in) to 58 cm (23 in) long with a good heat insulating layer of fat. Large areas of the body and scalp are often covered with vernix, a white substance like cream cheese. The skin may be mottled. It may have sideburns and hair low on the nape of the neck and sometimes down the back as well, which is not the hair that will remain, but is the remains of *lanugo*, which protected the skin in utero. Particularly if the child is premature there are likely to be large quantities of lanugo. It cries vigorously, grips tightly with both hands and feet, sucks energetically and can root around for the nipple. If the mother strokes at either side of the mouth it will turn and start searching for something to suck. Some babies are born sucking their thumbs or fingers; the majority who are not sleepy from the mother's anaesthetic will suck well if put to the breast immediately, once the air ways are completely clear. It takes about thirty breaths a minute, although this has not the steady rhythm of the older child and adult, and many mothers have lain awake at night listening to the odd noises their new babies make, quick pants, little snorts, followed by quick breathing again.

The baby can pass urine—and has been doing so in utero since early in pregnancy, and may do so as it is being born—and *meconium*, a greeny-black substance which forms the first contents of the bowel. If the child is distressed in labour, or if—because of a breech presentation—the trunk is getting very squashed as it is pressed first down the birth canal, it may pass this meconium even before delivery, and this means that the waters are stained. It is a danger signal for which labour attendants watch. The baby can yawn and sneeze and is capable even at this early age of a variety of facial expressions.

Parents who expected their infants to look like the babies in babyfood advertisements may find that their baby looks rather odd. It is a good idea for the antenatal teacher to prepare prospective parents for the common variations in the newborn baby. In doing this quotations from other new parents' impressions of their babies are very useful, ranging from the man who thought his violet and purple shaded baby looked, as it emerged from the birth canal, like 'a badly drawn ordnance survey map', to the one who reacted to the impact of his breech delivered son, 'He looked just like an oven-ready pheasant!'

'Babies may have little spots like minute pimples over the nose, cheeks and chin,' the teacher can explain. 'These form in the sweat glands, and disappear in the first week. Blotches on the eyelids and between the eyes, sometimes called *stork bites* are really pressure marks, and they disappear too.'

You will certainly need to discuss moulding of the head and the appearance of a caput, 'the part of the baby's head which was pressing down in the cervix', and you should explain that this soft blister-like protuberance goes in a couple of days. Cephalhaematoma should also be explained especially as this may not be obvious at delivery, and becomes obvious only on the second day and then becomes more pronounced for another day or so. By the end of a week the edges may calcify so that the parents can get the impression that the baby has a 'hole in the head'. Most haematomas disappear by six weeks, although a few take longer. Moulding can also occur to the face, causing a lop-sided look, and to the foot.

The size of the genitals may prove alarming to the parents, unless they realize that they look relatively large in a newborn baby, and especially in a premature baby. Sometimes in boys there is oedema of the scrotum as a result of pressure, but this goes down after a week or so. In baby girls the clitoris may look big and there may be a white vaginal discharge and sometimes blood. Both boys and girls may have slightly swollen breasts as a result of hormones in the mother's bloodstream which have passed through to the baby. Sometimes milk is produced, 'witch's milk', which should not be pressed out, but just left.

It should be explained that the immature liver may find it difficult to handle the bilirubin in the bloodstream, so that jaundice may result on the third or fourth day, which tends to make the baby less responsive and sleepier. These babies need a good deal of liquid, and should if necessary be woken for feeds. If jaundice is severe, photo-therapy treatment may be given to the baby.

In the uterus the baby has been lying curled up, and only gradually does it unfold from this womb position. Usually when it is put down to sleep for the first weeks it will assume the customary flexed position with knees drawn up and back rounded. Right from the beginning babies can creep and in an unassisted delivery may make creeping movements on emerging from the birth canal. This is a rudimentary form of crawling, and means that a baby who is put down on its front to sleep may quickly work its way up a carry cot until its head touches the top and after a few weeks there will be an obvious flattened bit of hair on the top of the head. If the baby is lying on the bed on its front and the mother or father presses a hand against the soles of the feet it may start to creep across the bed. The baby will also step out if held up, supported under the arms, with feet touching a firm surface. Moreover if bath sponge or book is put in front of one foot in the baby's progress forward, the other foot will automatically be lifted a little higher with the next step, as if to avoid the obstacle.

The baby hates being suddenly lowered, and shows a startle response if quickly lowered into a bath or almost dropped. This is called the *Moro response* and obviously has survival value; the arms are raised, the palms are brought together and the head jerks upward. Although a baby's head does not usually need supporting when simply being held, it does if the baby is being carried about or moved from one position to another and there is a chance of a sudden downward movement like this. Perhaps this is why some babies dis-like their baths; nervous handling may provoke the Moro response. On the other hand, new babies may also hate having all their clothes off and being unbound. Some babies startle even when their nappies are changed. They seem to like the firm holding provided by a firmly done up nappy.

At first the look the baby gives is very serious and intent, and, mother may think, rather critical. This can be a little disconcerting when one first puts a baby in the bath or changes its nappy. Babies can also follow a moving shape to which they are attracted, although they will 'lose' it easily and, because they have no experience, will not know where to pick it up visually again. Some babies hate bright light and are happiest in the old-fashioned cot with muslin or nylon curtains at the head end. Between eight and twelve weeks the baby discovers its hands as they pass its line of vision and will begin to acquire the coordination necessary to move these exciting objects in front of it and wave them about.

The baby hates loud sudden noises but likes music, the sound of a vacuum cleaner or washing machine, human voices, including the activity of other children playing nearby, and the ticking of clocks. Perhaps the clock ticking is reminiscent of the mother's heartbeat. Many babies will drop off to sleep better if they have a background of regular rhythmic sound, whether it is one of the Japanese records of a mother's heartbeats or simply a cheap alarm clock, or firm rhythmic patting of their bottoms. In the evening, when babies are often restless and fussing for two to three hours, during the first three months, television may prove interesting and soothing for short periods, and some parents listen to the record player while they cuddle the baby. There is nothing at all abnormal about a baby who requires handling in this way for a period each day, and it certainly does not mean that there is anything 'wrong with the milk'. It is not until two or three weeks that the baby begins to know its mother's voice, responds to it differently from other sounds, and seems to prefer it to other voices.

The Mother–Baby Relationship

All the newborn infant's skills are important for the kind of relationship it establishes with its caretakers. The baby is handed to the new mother and from that moment she starts to find out who this child is. A dialogue develops between the two which continues throughout the rest of their lives together in one form or another. A newborn baby is not just a sleeping, crying or sucking bundle, a passive little creature on which life acts, but in many ways already has a personality of its own, even though that character is only just budding. From birth the baby tackles its environment with highly specialized skills.* Many parents do not realize that their baby can see, for example, even if many things are a bit out of focus, and that from birth bright colours rather than wishy-washy primrose and pink and blue and patterns rather than plain surfaces are preferred. Babies may fix their eyes on the mother's or father's face when at first they are placed in their arms, looking intently into their eyes.

More and more is now being learned about the interaction of the baby with its parents. The one who is suffering from the effects of a difficult birth or who is drowsy from drugs, which the mother has received in labour and which have passed through her bloodstream to the baby, may be slow to breathe and cry at delivery and also may not be able to continue feeding for other than short periods of time and be sleepy during feeds, so that the mother has to work hard to keep it interested.† Moreover there seems to be less interaction between mother and baby, at least during the first ten days. This interaction, and the whole pattern of maternal behaviour towards the child, is very much affected by the type of delivery the woman had, the medication that was used, if any, whether the father was present, and the mother's relationship with her medical attendants.‡ It is a question not just of an infant's abilities but of the stimulus which is provided or which may be absent in the environment, and of the total pattern of relationships into which the baby is born. This is a whole new field of study in which we are beginning to look at babies in their social interaction from the very moment they are delivered.

A baby is not like a lump of clay which is moulded by society acting through its mother and father. It is born with inbuilt behavioural patterns which, in fact, tends to make its parent adapt to its basic needs. Because a baby spontaneously sucks in clusters, instead of all the time, for instance, there is a chance of the mother interacting with it in the pauses, and she often starts talking to her baby as

* Good material for the antenatal teacher can be found in Martin Bax and Judy Bernal, *Your Child's First Five Years* (London, Heinemann, 1974).

† See Martin Richards, 'The One-day-old Deprived Child', *New Scientist* (March 28, 1974).

‡ See Aidan Macfarlane, 'If a Smile Is So Important', *New Scientist* (April 25, 1974).

it stops and looks up at her. This is one way in which communication develops between them. When mothers talk to their babies like this they stop and wait for the baby to respond, and then the baby takes over and vocalizes in its turn, then pauses, and it is the mother's turn. It is the beginning of a true conversation. The teacher can point out that the mother who is observing her baby and really responding to it, rather than simply being the director, spontaneously synchronizes her behaviour with that of the baby. This is not yet a genuine social reciprocity 'but is entirely due to the mother letting herself be paced by the infant's periodic behaviour'.* And in the same way that synchrony occurs with talking, so it does visually, as when the baby's gaze directs the mother's attention to an object, who takes her cue from the baby's behaviour. The baby's vocalization and pauses and visual behaviour thus act as signals to the attentive mother and are the foundation of later social development.

Most mothers want to handle and explore their newborn babies as soon as possible, although in the strange and often intimidating atmosphere of hospital and in the presence of strangers, many need in effect to be 'given permission' to do so. A teacher may like to ask a class, How do you think you'll feel when the baby is just born? One subject which mothers want to discuss is whether they will be allowed to hold the baby immediately. From all the evidence available it looks as if it is important for the emotional bonding of mother and infant and the mother's self-confidence in her ability to mother that women be supported in knowing how to convey tactfully but unequivocally to delivery room staff that they want to have their babies with them and to be given ample opportunity to examine, stroke and cuddle them, and that if they wish to breastfeed they should be permitted to put them to the breast on the delivery table, and to have unlimited flesh-to-flesh contact.

* Rudolph Schaffer, 'Behavioural synchrony in infancy' *New Scientist* (April 4, 1974).

21

The Fourth Trimester

The delivery of a baby marks the end of pregnancy. But it is not only this. It is part of a continuum in the lives of the new parents, and involves change for every single member of the family into which the baby is born. Although birth is the dramatic crisis which terminates pregnancy, it also raises the curtain on a new drama for which many couples are ill-prepared, and one which can be turbulent, traumatic and long-lasting.

Preparation for birth, in focusing on the labour as the activity for which the expectant mother is being trained, can fragmentize the experience of childbearing and may even contribute to the feeling of complete let-down and failure after delivery. The party is over; the spotlights are dimmed. There is the frightening task of getting down to being a mother. Moreover, the father's necessary emotional adjustments are often forgotten. To educate women, and men too, to adjust to the demands of the postpartum period and, indeed, for parenthood and its never-ending crises, childbirth preparation needs to be a good deal more than a drill for coping with contractions. It should give opportunity for full and free discussion about the changed roles involved in becoming a mother and father, about the feelings we get when a baby cries—and goes on crying whatever we do, and how to adapt to the needs of a vociferous, squalling, strange, and often frankly unattractive intruder in the home.

There is a fourth trimester to pregnancy, and we neglect it at our peril. It is a transitional period of approximately three months after birth, particularly marked after first babies, when many women are emotionally highly vulnerable, when they experience confusion and recurrent despair, and during which anxiety is normal and states of reactive depression commonplace. During this postpartum phase the woman is learning how to be a mother, and is getting to know and understand her baby. Motherhood does not really consist in the skills of feeding, bathing and changing a baby, although it expresses itself through these tasks. It involves an image the woman has of herself in relation to the baby. If this is missing it is difficult for her to act with spontaneity, and every task becomes burdensome and exhausting.

Even women who have ample experience of other people's small babies—midwives and nurses for example—can encounter major difficulties during this period of adjustment, which has been called that of 'primary maternal preoccupation'.* It can be still more intense when the baby is premature, or handicapped in any way, or when the mother has not been encouraged to handle and explore the baby from the moment of birth onwards, and especially when she is denied access to the baby and prevented from caring for it and feeling that she has the right and the ability to do so.

Need for Loving Support

The fourth trimester is a time during which every woman needs continuing and loving support. Much more is at stake than simply her confidence in the maternal role. The relationship of mother and child, the marriage and the mental health of the family may be at risk. Birth occurs at the crossing-point of the generations. If we can help mothers, and fathers too, at the point when the new family is initiated we are taking on a challenge in preventive psychotherapy which can have benefits for the whole family.

Subclinical postnatal depression is probably much more common than is supposed. One highly experienced psychiatric social worker who only realized what had hit her when she began to climb out of it commented: 'I had come to the end of the lollipop, and all I had left was the stick.'

During pregnancy there is increasing identification with the baby

*D. W. Winnicott, *The Maturational Processes and the Facilitating Environment* (London, Hogarth, 1965).

in utero. In the last months the fetus is part of the mother's self, and birth can seem like an amputation. In reports of dreams during pregnancy many mothers tell of dreams of losing parts of themselves, a limb or teeth, or have dreams in which an amputation is performed. After delivery the new mother is suddenly confronted with the baby's surprising otherness, and has to come to terms with the child outside her, who may be very different from the fantasy baby.

The fantasy image was of an attractive, cuddly and, above all, sleeping baby. Yet the one she has to handle has a receding chin, a sloping forehead, a flattened nose, piggy eyes, blotches on its skin, a scrawny neck like a tortoise, large genitals, a weird cord stump, hair growing down over its back, and may not be of the sex she hoped for. It cries, and moreover, screams *at* her, telling her unmistakably that she has no right to be a mother. She has to cope with the death of the fantasy baby and to accept this alien baby. Thus even when a baby is live and healthy there may be an initial period extraordinarily like that of grieving for a lost or handicapped child.

Baby's Fierce and Relentless Demands

The newborn's animal nature can also come as a shock. The baby obviously does not speak the same language that civilized adults speak, and its demands are fierce and relentless. The mother easily feels resentment, irritation, even hatred, and then overpowering guilt that she experiences these 'unmaternal' reactions. This is because our society has sentimentalized motherhood and imbued it with a madonna-and-child sweetness which it is impossible for any flesh-and-blood woman to live up to.

In this state of confusion and guilt the new mother invariably receives advice from her mother and mother-in-law, from other women and from professionals, particularly if she is hoping to breastfeed. Much of this advice is contradictory and conflicting. Under these circumstances it can seem as if others are trying to take possession of the baby and asserting that she has no right to it, and she may temporarily develop paranoid fantasies.

Many women believe that sheer maternal instinct will bring love as soon as the little creature is put in their arms. For every mother the relationship with a new baby is of the nature of a love affair, and love affairs can vary widely. Some are a 'falling' in love, which takes place at first sight or sometimes much later; others are slow to grow and the realization of love gradually dawns.

Expectant parents need a chance to talk about these subjects and to hear other new parents' experiences and their emotional responses to the baby. It is important that couples should be invited to come back to preparation classes to talk about not only their experience of childbirth, but about the stresses, challenges, and joys of the immediate postpartum weeks.

Process of Bonding

During the first days and even in the first minutes after birth, the process of bonding begins to take place between all mammals and their young. A great deal can be done to help bonding between the parents and the new baby immediately after delivery if they are given ample opportunities for flesh-to-flesh contact, ideally in bed. If only hospitals could provide double beds big enough for mother and father and baby to cuddle together, just as they would at home. When the mother gets little chance to discover and get to know her baby in hospital the transition between hospital and home, the sudden handing over of the baby from the experts to the novice mother, can be very disturbing.

Where mothers, and fathers too when they are free to be there, can themselves care for the baby even while mother and her baby are still in hospital, and enjoy it together without feeling incompetent, the gulf between hospital and home is less abrupt. Yet it is not only for the baby's sake that a couple need to be alone together with their baby. It is important for the marriage too. For they need to be able to see, approve of and discover each other anew in their roles as parents.

In the intensity of the mother-neonate relationship the new father can quickly feel superfluous, and an intruder not only in the hospital but in his own home. Then to both man and woman the arrival of the baby can seem to threaten their romance, and the seeds of marriage problems are sown which develop into destructive marital crises over the years. When they have a chance to learn care of the baby together, to experiment, make mistakes and learn at their own pace, the man rarely feels that he is being pushed out of the picture or that he is unwanted. From the moment that a baby enters a marriage the way in which the man and woman act and react to each other in their roles as parents, and the aspects of each other's personalities that are revealed in parenthood, are elements as vital in their relationship as sex, money or the in-laws.

The process of adjustment is often a tiring one for both of them. Yet it is the woman who is with the baby all day, often virtually imprisoned in the house and isolated from all her usual social contacts. She waits for the man's return from work, bringing a breath of the outside world, the real life of action, amusing conversation, scintillating discussion, perhaps. There is a step at the door and in he comes, tired, his face drawn and pale, brow puckered with worry, and her hopes are dashed. It is easy to forget that the new father is likely to be tired too, not just from broken nights but from having to adjust to a completely new role. We have responsibilities to the marriage into which a baby is born, and those in maternity care should see their functions as extending to prenatal preparation and, where necessary, postnatal support of the *couple*, not only as parents, but as husband and wife, through this difficult transitional period of the fourth trimester.

Coming to Terms with Body Changes

During this time too the woman needs to come to terms with her changed body. Immediately after birth there is often a sense of emptiness and she can hardly realize that the baby is in fact outside her body. Yet she is not as she was before the pregnancy. She is faced with pads soaking with blood, sweat, colostrum, engorged breasts, sticky milk oozing out all over the place and a crumpled, flabby abdomen. She has probably had an episiotomy and is worried that love-making will never be the same again.

Moreover, in the care she is given it seems that her body has been taken over by the hospital and is no longer her own. Prodded and poked, injected, strapped, moved into position, linked up to monitoring devices, palpated, explored vaginally, hoisted into lithotomy, given suppositories or an enema, cut off from all or part of her physical sensations by anaesthesia, looked at critically, assessed and examined, her body is no longer the seat of sensory delight but is completely alien. It is not surprising that postnatal frigidity is a common experience nor, since the two are linked, that postnatal impotence on the part of the man is a not infrequent occurrence.

However, it is not just that the woman's body can seem so strange to her. When she is concentrating on the baby she is unable to focus attention on pleasurable physical sensations. There is nothing more inhibiting than listening to a new baby's breathing or waiting for its urgent cry of hunger when making love.

In many ways primitive and peasant societies seem to manage the transitional period into motherhood rather better than we do. Although the new mother may go straight back to hoeing the fields and stirring the cooking pot, the postpartum period is ritually defined, and she is considered to be in a *marginal* state of being.

In my anthropological field work in Jamaica I observed that newly delivered women kept their heads wrapped in turbans to protect them from 'baby chill', often burned incense to attract the 'good angels', avoided washing their hair for something like forty days after birth, and were very careful not to see a dead body. Ritual avoidance may persist for days, weeks, or months after birth. At the same time the situation is not static; rites act as signposts through what we might consider as the transitional process, each ceremony both marking the gateway through which the mother and child, and often other members of the family, are passing and pointing towards the next. Although these ceremonial rites centre on the child they always involve change and often increased social status for the mother, and sometimes for both parents.

Because they also draw in members of the extended family and other kinsmen, as well as neighbours, and often invoke the help of ancestors, the ceremonies also have the effect of reinforcing social solidarity, and unity both of the living and the dead in support of the new mother. Religious observances, feasting and merry-making celebrate the change in the parents' status.

Period of Recurring Crisis

Psychologically in our own society this fourth trimester is one of recurring crisis. Yet it is in no way a sign of mental illness and can be considered a normal life crisis. Sometimes, however, there is obvious disproportionate anxiety or depression, or the state continues well beyond the first fourteen weeks. Only when the woman completely denies or rejects her baby in the postpartum weeks, or when four or five months after the birth her whole life still revolves around the baby, so that anxiety is interfering with her 'becoming herself 'again, can we be sure that it is pathological.

Through this crisis period women *need* support. Some may wish their own mothers to be actively involved in this, although in the case of the infantile primipara, who is overdependent on her mother, this is not the wisest solution. Many women today prefer to look to emotional support from other women who are going through or who have recently passed through the same experience. It is, in a way, support from sisters. Some antenatal teachers working with the National Childbirth Trust have been helping with the setting up of peer groups who learn how to give active support and friendship to women after childbirth.

These postnatal support groups function not primarily to help women with the practical tasks of baby care and with breastfeeding problems, although these are often discussed, but to offer emotional support and simple counselling to women who may be feeling socially isolated, anxious and depressed. Helpers need to be available on the telephone day and night and to be ready to go into a woman's home if necessary. In the case of the group working in Oxford and area they function very closely with the community midwives and are often introduced to a mother who is going through a period of stress by the midwife dealing with the case, who may take the member of the support group to the distressed woman's home so that they can meet. It is emphasized that this kind of help does not conflict with the help given by the health visitor, but is the sort of friendship which exists side by side with it. Members of the group sit in on antenatal classes, and every class member is given a card with the name and address of the group member she can contact if she needs someone to talk to.

The physical or emotional battering of a baby does not suddenly begin in a parent who previously only had beautiful and loving thoughts about that child. Hostility towards a baby often grows out of great personal distress and an unhappy marriage. We should not wait until parents are actually assaulting their children before we come in to offer help and friendship. Postnatal support groups provide one of the most hopeful ways in which the challenge of the fourth trimester can be met.

22

Postnatal Depression

Some teachers shy away from talking about depression after child-birth, because they wonder if such discussion may not actually increase the chances of it occurring. Others talk about it as if it happened to everybody, as inevitably following birth as night follows day. Neither is a realistic approach to the subject. The emotions of the postpartum period are all part of the fascinating adventure of child-birth, and whatever form they take, are as integral to the story as are the dilatation of the cervix and rotation of the fetal head.

The teacher does not have to say, Now we will talk about depression, slotting it into a syllabus along with the third stage and breastfeeding, but should have her antennae out to respond to any readiness in the group to discuss together postpartum emotional changes. If such discussion is not forthcoming, she may choose to initiate it by saying something like, Have you thought about how you may feel the day after the baby is born? . . . three days after? . . . three weeks after? Those of you who have friends or sisters who have had babies fairly recently, have they told you how they felt then? . . . and so on.

Probably two-thirds of new mothers have some depression after childbirth. Often this is only the sudden tearfulness connected with endocrine changes, which is similar to the premenstrual tension with which many women are familiar. Enough people experience it to say that it is normal, and does not mean that a mental illness is starting. This is so even though nearly half these women not only feel desperately miserable but are disturbed to find they cannot think coherently.

Depression is common on the third or fourth day, when it is often called *the baby blues*, but often it is not realized that they can occur in the next few weeks as well. This minor reactive depression seems to happen more often to women having hospital rather than home confinements, especially if they are parted from the baby because it is kept in the nursery for a time. So is it particularly likely to occur after a labour which was difficult for the baby, or when the baby was premature. It is also more likely to happen with a woman who has always had violent mood swings, whether or not she has just had a baby.

The third or fourth day blues are partly a reaction similar to that after any exciting and dramatic event. Birth is the climax of pregnancy. The teacher can say that many women suffer a tremendous feeling of let-down and anticlimax after the hoping, waiting and planning, the hard work of labour, and the thrilling delivery of the baby. Now the 'party' is over, and there seems nothing left to look forward to. But there is more to it than that.

A new mother is different from the woman she was before the birth. She often feels she is acting a part which is not really hers. This can be intensified by being in the unfamiliar environment of hospital and being treated as a sick person.

Depression in the early days can be part of a stressful relationship with nurses and midwives. Sometimes their efficiency in coping with the baby may seem to the new mother who is lacking in confidence—and probably most are—that another woman is trying to take her baby away from her, and could develop into paranoid feelings which involve a conviction that this person is out to harm the baby or herself. Women often reenact a difficult relationship with their own mothers in their relations with women caring for them in childbirth as if the mother feels that she may have no right to the baby, and that she has stolen it from her mother, or from the nurse who represents her mother. It is only by having the chance to get to know her baby and to care for it herself that a mother begins to cope with this sort of stress.

However, it is not only this kind of fantasy which contributes to the new mother's vulnerability. In the early postpartum days it is as she were on the margins between two states of existence, a bridge between two identities. We have noted already that primitive societies recognize this and have special rites to protect the mother and child in this 'no man's land' between birth and ordinary living.

When this sort of depression is experienced later than a few days after the birth but still within the next few weeks, or when it recurs during this time, it may be that the new mother is still in a transitional state. It is as if she needs time to mourn the loss of herself as she was before she became a mother, or sometimes to mourn the loss of 'the doll in the toy cupboard', the idealized image of the baby while it was still in the womb, who is now revealed as a squalling infant with a blotchy skin and a receding brow and chin.

When she is home again and taking responsibility for the baby, fatigue also plays a part. The baby's constant demands can be exhausting, and every action that will later become familiar routine and be performed casually, she thinks about and analyses—and then perhaps goes back and does it all again in case she did not do it right the first time. She listens to the baby screaming, and feels frustration, resentment, despair, and often sheer hatred, and then a great wave of guilt sweeps over her because she feels all these things. The yelling stops, and she rushes in to see if the baby has died and wakes it up! She worries about the odd sounds of baby's breathing as it sleeps, with quick little breaths and then a sigh, and perhaps a little crow. Is it getting pneumonia? She wonders if it is warm enough, or too hot. A sticky eye, common in newborn babies, seems a major infection. Small weight gains lead her to feel that the baby is wasting away and, if she is breastfeeding, that she is unworthy to be a mother, and she weeps in despair.

All the time she is doing this she is sending out signals to the baby about her distress and tension. Often the baby understands non-verbal language very well, arches its back and refuses to feed, startles easily, will not settle when put down to sleep, and seems to get as irritable and jumpy as she is. Meanwhile the anxious mother shuts her husband out in the cold and immerses herself in the baby and its needs, with which she totally identifies herself.

The anxiety which may accompany the state of concentrated

attention on the baby, or Winnicott's *primary maternal preoccupation*, normally lasts for anything up to eight weeks after the birth of a first baby. It is unlikely to occur with second and subsequent babies. It merges with depression, for there is really no hard and fast line between anxiety and depression in the first postpartum weeks. The teacher can explain that it is part of learning to be a mother, and is a sort of growing pain.

Depression of this kind is usually simply a sign that the new mother is having to make difficult emotional adjustments. It does no good at all to tell her to pull herself together! So when she is tired or irritable, when she is aggressive with her mother, her mother-in-law or the health visitor, if she flies off the handle at the least thing, loses all interest in sex, and will not stop worrying about the baby, the first thing a husband needs to remember is to avoid criticism and cheerful pep talks. He should let her know that he loves her, that he has faith in her as a mother, and, protecting her from all the well-meant advice that pours in, offer a strong shoulder to cry on.

For many mothers there has to be something like a second birth when they move a little away from the baby emotionally and are ready to be not only mothers but themselves again, for at least part of the time. A woman cannot forever live in and through her child. The emotional umbilical cord must be severed and the child, too, allowed to be himself or herself. Gradually the husband can take over some caring for the baby, and can see that his wife gets out and away from the child for at least short periods.

One of the greatest challenges of parenthood, which applies to fathers as well as to mothers, is that parents should not be simply caretakers, but people who go on growing.

Breakdown

Some women experience postnatal depression merged with anxiety very severely, go through a phase when they feel they cannot cope at all, and are recognizably at the end of their tether. If the doctor sees them he may diagnose it as neurotic depression. It is not completely different from the more often encountered anxiety mixed with depression, but is further along the scale of distress.

It is more likely to occur with painful severity in our society when a woman is very dependent on her mother and lacks confidence in her ability to be a mother, or even sometimes a separate person, herself. It is associated, too, with an obsessional striving to live up to standards which are impossible to meet.

Sometimes, for example, the woman has a rigid picture of the person she wants to be and what she is aiming at in her life, and the baby plays no part in this, or, like most babies, does not behave in a convenient or a predictable way. Life then becomes a struggle between ideal and reality, and between the baby and the mother, from early morning to the middle of the night. A woman who has had a successful career and who cannot adapt herself to the baby sometimes faces this sort of depression. She sees other women around her who seem to be managing much better than she is, and this only increases her despair. She is not only anxious about everything she does for the baby but often terrified that she is going to hurt it or do something terrible, like drowning it in the bath water. If she is not given loving emotional support, each day may take on a nightmare quality of dread that she is going to harm the child. As if to safeguard herself from this terror, some depressed women just 'blot out' the baby, and seem completely indifferent to it. It is as if they are so frightened of what they might do that the safest way is to deny the child's existence.

Occasionally the woman becomes very confused and disoriented, not knowing whether it is day or night, for instance, and may feel that the only way out is suicide, and there is a real risk that she may do so. This is mental illness, and skilled help, drugs and psychotherapy are needed. The teacher or other postnatal counsellor must make it clear that *the husband should not wait for his wife to agree to see the doctor*, but should go himself to ask the doctor to visit, and say that a psychiatric consultation would be welcome.

A woman can put off seeking help either because of a total inertia or because she and her husband are ashamed to acknowledge the need for expert guidance, or sometimes because she feels everyone is against her. There is no reason to think that, given help of this kind, she may not after a few months to a year or so, again be living a useful and positive life.

Another kind of breakdown is called *puerperal psychosis*. It rarely comes out of the blue. In a way it is only indirectly connected with the birth, and might equally well take place in adolescence, at the menopause or at any other major change in one's life. The mother loses touch with reality; there seems no connection between the person she once was and the woman she is now; she may have hallucinations. Sometimes she wants to kill her baby or believes that it has died. The woman who has had a previous mental illness of this kind is more at risk than one who has never suffered one before. In this case it is important for her to have psychiatric help during the pregnancy, and the psychiatrist may start medication before the baby is born, while she is still feeling quite herself, so greatly reducing the chance of a breakdown after.

Whatever kind of depression a woman suffers from it may be a necessary stage of emotional growth which has to be passed through in one way or another for that particular woman. Christian in *The Pilgrim's Progress* had to go on past the Slough of Despond. He could not pretend that it did not exist, or go another way, or stop short when he encountered it. There are many women who have been through severe depression who can look back on it from the standpoint of a new serenity and maturity.

If a new mother is depressed the chances are that she is not embarked on a mental illness, but that it is an emotional growing pain. However well-organized and happy other women seem, most have the same doubts and worries as she does. There is no quick remedy, no miracle drug for the suffering that is involved in growing up, and having a baby is a good time for growing up.

23

Helping Through the Experiences of Miscarriage and Stillbirth

I carried you in hope,
the long nine months of my term,
remembered that close hour when we made you,
often felt you kick and move
as slowly you grew within me,
wondered what you would look like
when your wet head emerged,
girl or boy, and at what glad moment
I should hear your birth cry,
and I welcoming you
with all you needed of warmth and food;
we had a home waiting for you.

After my strong labourings,
sweat cold on my limbs,
my small cries merging with the summer air,
you came. You did not cry.
You did not breathe.
We had not expected this;
it seems your birth had no meaning,
or had you rejected us?

They will say that you did not live,
register you as still-born.

> But you lived for me all that time
> in the dark chamber of my womb;
> and when I think of you now,
> perfect in your little death,
> I know that for me you are born still;
> I shall carry you with me for ever,
> my child, you were always mine,
> you are mine now.

> Death and life are the same mysteries.*

MISCARRIAGE

About 10 to 25 per cent of babies are spontaneously aborted before the twenty-eighth week of pregnancy, the majority in the first twelve weeks. It is impossible to be accurate because many women lose their babies before they know they are pregnant, and simply have what seems to be a late period.

In approximately 66 per cent of cases these are the babies who would not have developed perfectly; the earlier any abnormality develops in the embryo, when initial cell division is taking place, and a little later when the main body structures like the heart, brain and digestive system are forming, the more severe that abnormality is likely to be. So it is these babies who might have been gravely damaged if they had survived till birth.

Most women probably do not need or want counselling, and manage to cope with the experience of miscarriage. At the same time, there are frequently dark moments—often in the middle of the night—and it is then particularly that a woman tends to look for causes of the miscarriage and to explain it by remembering that she slipped and fell on the stairs or that she had intercourse the night before, that she got worked up about her mother-in-law coming to stay, or had a shock when she saw someone knocked off his bicycle by a passing car. She probably does this because as we know from ways in which witchcraft functions in primitive societies,† it helps

* The poem *Stillborn* by Leonard Clark is printed by special permission of the poet.

† See E. E. Evans-Pritchard: *Witchcraft, Oracles and Magic Among the Azande* (London, O.U.P., 1937).

psychologically to be able to relate catastrophes to a specific ascertainable cause. On the whole contemporary medical opinion is that although environmental stress can affect uterine function through the secretion of hormones, such incidents rarely cause miscarriage. The counsellor may explain that the cause is more likely to be that there was abnormal development of the fetus, or in the remaining cases, where the fetus was normal, that the woman ran a very high temperature with an infection, or that there was something inhospitable about the lining of the uterus in which, the counsellor can say, the fetus embeds itself rather like a plant with its roots in the soil.

In about eight out of ten cases of bleeding in early pregnancy, especially if the bleeding is slight, the pregnancy continues smoothly afterwards, and the mother bears a healthy baby. Antenatal teachers need to know this and to be able to give expectant mothers the information. In fact some slight spotting of blood at the time when the first couple of periods were due is very common, and although it may be a good idea for the woman to rest in bed until it clears up and to take life more gently for the next few weeks, bleeding of this kind does not suggest that she needs medical care or drugs; it is, rather, an indication that she should learn how to relax completely, physically, mentally and emotionally.

When bleeding continues and increases, and is accompanied by cramp-like pain similar to that of a painful period, abortion is said to be inevitable, and in that case the sooner it takes place, the better. In all cases of bleeding at any stage of pregnancy the expectant mother should let her doctor know immediately.

Most miscarriages take place within the first three months, but when bleeding occurs between the twelfth and twenty-eighth weeks of pregnancy the cause is more likely to be that the cervix is weak, and then repeated miscarriages may be experienced.

The teacher can tell the expectant mother that even if a woman has had a previous miscarriage there is an 80 per cent chance that her next pregnancy will be uneventful. This is slightly reduced if she has already had two successive miscarriages, but she still has a 75 per cent chance of a live, healthy baby; and even if she has had three successive miscarriages she has a 70 per cent chance that it will not happen again.

Whatever the statistical chances of bearing a live baby next time, most women find a miscarriage distressing. The impact is usually less marked within the first three months, before a woman has really adjusted to her pregnancy and has felt movement, but it often causes grief and mourning for the lost baby after that time. She often feels this much more keenly than her husband, who sometimes finds her sorrow irritating, and, although he wants to sympathize, is embarrassed by what he sees as excessive grief. He may be told by friends to jolly her out of it with a holiday or by going out, and trying to cheer her up generally. And certainly this may work. But if she is depressed she cannot simply 'snap out of it'.

Many husbands are bewildered by mourning of this kind, seek escape from it in preoccupation with work, or in social relationships, and then feel guilty that they are not able to demonstrate the sympathy and understanding which they feel their wives are demanding. This is one reason why miscarriage, and especially a series of miscarriages, can be a serious stress for the marriage. The man, too, may feel responsible, and even though he knows rationally that he did not cause the loss of the baby, may feel that if only he were a better husband this would not have happened. Feelings of this kind are sometimes the beginning of a long path of recrimination, misunderstandings and resentment.

The man may suffer in other ways, too, after a miscarriage. When it looked as if the woman he loved—but with whom there were stormy emotional scenes—might lose her baby, one unmarried man said, 'This will finish me, and it will finish our relationship'. The birth of a live child would be proof of his virility and masculinity, and the loss of that child threatened him with emasculation. The woman in this case was not only going to lose her baby, but her man too.

Counselling by the general practitioner, a psychotherapist, or the antenatal teacher can often help after a miscarriage. In some cases, where there are psychosomatic causes for miscarriage, this can have primary therapeutic value, and Llewelyn-Jones believes that 'this is most clearly seen in the patient who habitually aborts, and the only common factor in the success of the many treatments offered is the interest shown in the patient by the obstetrician'.*

Some women become anxious and protective about their bodies, keenly aware of all physical sensations, and so disappointed as each menstrual period comes that they feel the inconvenience and the discomfort of the contracting uterus much more intensely than before. Each period then becomes for them a sort of miscarriage, and with the first signs of bleeding they mourn again yet another lost baby. Some react hysterically; that is, they have physical illnesses which are psychosomatic in origin.

One of these hysterical illnesses is *pseudocyesis*, or phantom pregnancy. The woman misses her periods, sometimes for months on end, swells up, and often has nausea and vomiting and other signs of pregnancy, but is really not pregnant at all. She is not pretending; she honestly believes she is pregnant. In other cases there may be a severe emotional imbalance, linked with the painful feelings of loss, which lead a woman to take another woman's baby. What she is suffering then corresponds to puerperal depression, but in this case depression is centred on the actual experience of loss.

Even where a couple go on living an apparently normal life and the woman is coping well with the miscarriage, there can be strains on a marriage because they feel they have to prove themselves reproductively capable. Often when a woman has miscarried there has been an event in her previous history to which she can look back as possibly causing the disaster: an attack of venereal disease years before or an induced abortion in adolescence before she knew her husband and which she may not have told him about; such things can weigh heavily on her mind.

The woman may start taking her temperature every morning to discover when she is ovulating. She may be insistent about having intercourse just at that time, when he may not feel particularly interested. A man can soon begin to feel that he is being used like a stud bull. Such concentration of purpose on intercourse at the time of ovulation is often linked with lack of interest in intercourse at other times, especially in the last half of the menstrual cycle, when

* Derek Llewelyn-Jones, *Fundamentals of Obstetrics & Gynecology*, Vol. I, *Obstetrics* (London, Faber, 1973).

she thinks she may be pregnant and he is nervous about dislodging the embryo. Intercourse then becomes a planned mechanical exercise, and changes from love-making into a test of reproductive ability. The passion of lovers is lost in the passion for a baby. This stress on the marriage may cause it to reach breaking point within a couple of years of the baby's birth, when the mother is engrossed in the child and its need of her, and the husband is pushed increasingly into the background.

The counsellor can say that unless there is continued or intermittent bleeding during pregnancy, or bleeding follows intercourse, love-making can continue throughout the nine months. If there has been a previous miscarriage, it may be wise to avoid intercourse during those days when the periods would have been due during the second and third months. Gentle, considerate and tender love-making can be an excellent thing for the woman's peaceful, happy state of mind, and for reminding her of what complete relaxation feels like. If she is trying to 'hold on' to her pregnancy, the very tension may contribute towards the tendency to miscarry.

The counsellor can stress that after a miscarriage, loving, tender care is the best medicine. Because the whole of life shrinks under the impact of grief, stimulus, judiciously applied, is necessary: a change of scene, perhaps, a task in which she is able to get involved without concentrating all her thoughts on her loss, fresh interests, and emotional support which can help her feel valued as a person. This is important because after a miscarriage one feels a failure *as a woman*, and anything that the husband does to make her feel desired and valued can gradually give her back her confidence in herself.

It is usually a good idea to wait to conceive again until the woman is feeling fit; although this must be qualified as some women do not feel themselves again until they know they are pregnant once more. The counsellor may suggest that the intervening weeks or months need not be wasted, and she can build up her general health by diet, two or three very early nights each week, and by learning how to relax. The antenatal teacher may be able to set aside time to give the woman who has had a series of miscarriages some lessons in relaxation of body *and mind*.

When the next pregnancy starts the doctor or antenatal teacher may suggest that special arrangements should be made for more rest. Sometimes a job proves exhausting and it is wise to seek leave of absence in the first weeks. Long journeys are best avoided and if lengthy car journeys are necessary, the driver should stop every hour or so and let the pregnant woman get out and walk around. As an extra safety measure the counsellor may advise the pregnant woman to avoid all drugs, including cigarettes and alcohol, although an occasional glass of wine may help her 'unwind'. Occasionally the gynaecologist decides that a suture around the cervix, which hangs down into the vagina, like the mouth of a Victorian string bag, will help avoid cervical incompetence. He threads a loop around the incompetent cervix and draws it tight. This is then taken out just before the expected date of delivery, and labour frequently starts afterwards. This is used when the pregnancy was interrupted after the first weeks, and when the weight of the developing fetus and the stretching of the uterus caused the cervix to sag open.

When a woman has had a previous ectopic pregnancy, treatment has entailed cutting out the damaged section of the Fallopian tube affected. The patient will have been told that fortunately she has another tube the other side of the uterus, and although ova cannot travel along the tube on which surgery has been performed, they are able to do so the other side. After an operation of this kind the ovary often steps up production so that a ripe ovum is released into the remaining uterine tube every month.

In a pregnancy following a late miscarriage or a series of repeated miscarriages, at whatever stage of pregnancy they occurred, there is an advantage in offering the woman a private session in which the emphasis is put on relaxation and good body mechanics, and in which she is also given the opportunity to talk about her feelings. Miscarriage can be a very lonely experience, and if the baby is lost there is no product of the pregnancy to mourn. The counsellor can give emotional support by creating and maintaining an atmosphere in which the woman can 'reveal and recognize'* herself, accepting the reality of her experience of loss. Sometimes a counsellor finds it difficult to accept this reality when the miscarriage

* Michael and Enid Balint, *Psychotherapeutic Techniques in Medicine* (London, Tavistock Social Science Paperback, 1972).

occurred early in pregnancy. 'After all, it is not like losing a baby.' Balint has this to say about the counsellor's refusal to face the patient's reality:

If . . . a patient complains of abdominal pain, the doctor will not say, 'How awful, I can't stand you with these pains, go away to another doctor'; neither will he reassure the patient, 'Never mind, it is not so bad and, in any case, I will have sympathy and affection for you'; still less will he side-step or disregard the symptom. What he will do is to accept it and to examine it as well as he is able to.

When a woman becomes pregnant after a previous miscarriage, it is important that the teacher helps her acquire skills which will stand her in good stead whether or not the pregnancy continues, and is ready also to listen and understand her doubts, her feelings of guilt, the problems that may crop up in her marriage, and her apprehension about the future, all of which are mixed with her joy at finding herself again pregnant.

STILLBIRTH

Kate's baby was born dead. I did not meet her till some months after, when she was suffering from depression. She said she felt rejected by the group of mothers at classes with whom she had shared her pregnancy and also by her antenatal teacher, not because she was unsympathetic but because she had never gave her a chance to come and talk about the experience. The birth not only involved losing the baby but was an abrupt amputation from all the relationships she had formed during pregnancy. I talked to her teacher about it and found that it seemed to her inappropriate to ask Kate to come because she felt she had no specific skills for helping through this difficult situation, and thought it might be too painful for her to meet again the women whom she associated with her pregnancy. Whereas when everything went right and there was a happy labour and a beautiful, healthy baby, the mother came back to class and proudly reported on her labour as a great success story, in contrast the bereaved woman felt not only grief-stricken and unwanted but an utter failure.

A psychiatrist who wanted to do research on the emotional aspects of stillbirth wrote to a number of obstetricians to find out which of their patients had lost babies and how the women had coped with this experience. Time and time again he found that they did not know because they had not been in touch with the patient, or if they had, discussion on the subject had been brief and superficial. So he decided instead to have a look at how *doctors* coped with the experience of stillbirth, and discovered that they were, almost without exception, avoiding contact with their bereaved patients and keeping themselves as far removed as possible from a disagreeable matter. The doctor, as well as the woman, had a problem, and he concludes:

The doctor whose patient has had a stillbirth does not want to know, he does not want to notice and he does not want to remember anything about it. This must mean doctors under strain and a group of patients in danger of neglect.*

There is, in the words of another psychiatrist working on the subject, 'a conspiracy of silence.'†

The doctor's response is part of a much more general pattern of avoidance of grief among hospital staff. The person who is mourning is an embarrassment and almost an outcast. Outside hospitals, too, we tend to treat grief as if it were a highly contaminating and shameful sickness, so that the bereaved person has to apologize for her grief. Even when we want to help we are perplexed about what to say and how to behave. This is because their emotions are threatening to *us* and perhaps because those in the helping professions often cannot help feeling guilty, as if they had somehow caused the death.

One way of handling the anxiety surrounding childbirth is that of denial and 'magical repair'. Hospital staff tell the mother: Don't let yourself dwell on it. . . . Be brave! . . . Think about something else. . . . Pull yourself together! . . . Put it behind you! or Have another

* S. Bourne's paper entitled 'The Psychological Effects of Stillbirth on the Doctor' is in *Psychosomatic Medicine in Obstetrics and Gynaecology*, N. Morris, ed. (Basel, Karger, 1972).

† A. E. Lewis, 'Reactions to Stillbirth' in N. Morris, ed., *ibid.*

baby!; or they may keep her heavily sedated for their own comfort.* Where the baby is living, but grossly handicapped and unlikely to survive, many hospitals take over total care of the child themselves, make all the important decisions about it with minimal consultation with the parents, and as a matter of policy keep the mother away from her baby, presumably with the idea that this will save her pain. But it is by no means always the case that to avoid seeing or handling the baby somehow makes the situation less stressful, and it is important that there is flexibility in hospital arrangements for those mothers who do want to get to know their babies to do so. As one mother, who had been delivered of a baby with a large occipital encephalecele, put it:

I was luckier than many mothers of defective babies, my baby lived three weeks and I had an opportunity to get to know her—the real of her. How could I face myself now if I had followed the doctors' advice that I disassociate myself from her? Perhaps those who tried to protect me from facing reality thought the experience of pregnancy and birth could be erased by choice and by avoiding the child.†

Bereaved women who have been delivered in hospitals where open grief reactions are taboo, where they must suppress their feelings, or where these feelings are denied by simply ignoring them, exhibit symptoms of grief much longer than where it is accepted that initially the mother may need to pour out her pain, bewilderment—Why did this have to happen to *me*?—and hostility. In one Swedish hospital, of eleven women who suppressed their feelings seven were still showing mental symptoms of grieving after three months, whereas of forty-five women who openly expressed their feelings, only twelve were still grief-stricken beyond three months.‡

Sometimes reaction to loss of a loved person or object can be disproportionate, and then it does seem to become an illness. Although even then perhaps all we are saying is that the grief is more than that

*J. Cullberg, 'Mental Reactions of Women to Perinatal Death' in N. Morris, ed., *ibid.*

† Elizabeth Donnelly, The Real of Her', *J. of Obstetrics, Gynecologic and Neonatal Nursing*, Vol. III, No. 3 (May/June 1974).

‡ Cullberg, 'Mental Reactions of Women to Perinatal Death.'

particular society will tolerate. A widow throwing herself on her husband's funeral pyre would seem out of place in England, and Queen Victoria's long mourning for Albert would attract the attention of psychiatrists today.

The various forms of grieving have been divided into categories, and are described as *chronic* grief, *inhibited* grief and *delayed* grief. Chronic grief is an abnormal prolongation of grieving, with attacks of anxiety two or more years after the precipitating loss. In inhibited grief the person may express nothing. It is unresolved and waiting for expression, and eventually finds a way out in neurotic or psychosomatic illness or deep depression, a grieving characteristic of children who have suffered maternal deprivation. When grief is delayed it may find expression as mourning for a minor loss, while really the grief is centred on a major loss which occurred beforehand. When one woman's husband died from a coronary she went on living sensibly, without giving way to tears; but six months later her dog was run over, and she was suddenly overwhelmed with grief.*

In offering friendship to someone who is grieving we cannot come in, put things right, and take over the grief for them. Nor is it helpful to say, I know *just* what it's like, equate their present experience with grieving one has been through oneself, and somehow deny them the right to their *own* experience. We can only stand *beside* the bereaved person and 'share the grief work', without ourselves collapsing under its burden. We have, in fact, to 'honour' grief.† Whereas pretending not to notice or denying grief is unhelpful, insisting that a person express herself emotionally is an invasion of personality. People need their defences. We have no right to demand emotional collapse of anyone, and it is a very dangerous kind of interference. Real help lies somewhere *between* 'frontal assault'—a demand that the bereaved person break down and

* Murray Parkes, 'Grief as an Illness,' *New Society* (April, 1964). See also, 'Effects of Bereavement on Physical and Mental Health—A Study of the Medical Records of Widows,' *Br. med. J.*, 2:274 (1964).

† Robert B. Reeves, Jr, 'The Hospital Chaplain Looks at Grief', in Bernard Schoenberg and others, *Loss and Grief: Psychological Management in Medical Practice* (New York, Columbia University Press, 1970).

cry and express all the pent-up misery—on the one hand, and avoidance and denial of grief, on the other.

When there is an opportunity to prepare for loss it is less likely to be emotionally catastrophic. If a stillbirth, for example, is highly likely, it may be much better to give the parents some prior indication of difficulty than to whisk the little body away and then tell them that their baby is dead. Some doctors and midwives think it unnecessary and cruel to give the mother warning, especially when she still has the hard work of labour to do. It makes a difference when the relationship between the couple is strong and when the husband is helping his wife in childbirth, for then the grief, too, can be shared. Even so, some women in labour, even without their husbands with them, are perfectly aware that there is concern about the baby, even when staff think they have not let them know (and a great many more women *feel* that doctors and nurses are alarmed when in fact everything is going well). When husband and wife are close, and the preparation for birth has itself been shared, they can together start the work of anticipatory grieving, and this may cut down the duration and intensity of grieving when the actual crisis of stillbirth is reached.

Antenatal teachers often feel inhibited in offering support to the woman who has had a stillbirth because they have not been through the identical experience. But it is not necessary to have suffered the same loss in order to give help. Imaginative empathy is far more important than having had the same thing happen to you. To be able to do this we need to understand the many ways in which grief is expressed. It is easy to forget, for example, that hostility is an integral part of the grieving process. Friends of a bereaved woman often find it easier to support her when she is collapsed and weeping than when she is starting to fight back and be angry. But it is then too that she needs understanding.

The couple may want to talk through what has happened with doctors to find out exactly what happened, and what the prognosis is for any future pregnancy. Since, as we have seen, many doctors themselves retreat from this confrontation with grief, the teacher may be able to suggest ways in which appropriate action can be taken towards such discussion. In this, while acknowledging the bereaved person's anger, we must carefully avoid colluding with any irrational accusations about the care received.

Not only is it normal during the grieving process for a woman to express doubts about the medical care received but, perhaps, even more women blame *themselves* for things done or undone which they feel may have caused the baby's death. There is also a generalized feeling of emptiness, diminution of self, and failure, which is physically based and associated with the loss of the baby which was known so intimately in its intrauterine existence as well as with puerperal changes, the most pronounced of which may be the engorgement and discomfort of breasts preparing to lactate. There may be 'a deep feeling of physical inadequacy' which causes the woman to feel that she has been punished and deserves further punishment, often in the form of genital injury.*

At the same time the fact of having lost a baby is socially embarrassing. Acquaintances ask, What did you have? A boy or a girl? How's the baby? What happened? Where is it? and a woman can feel deeply ashamed when she has to confess that she has lost the child. She has become a 'non-mother'.

The father is often forgotten. He is almost invariably grieving too and yet feels less justified in giving way to grief. Moreover, in Anglo-Saxon culture, with its taboo on tenderness, men are not supposed to express emotions which suggest that they are soft or effeminate.

Often, too, there is another child to consider, the older sibling who has been deprived of an expected baby brother or sister. All children have destructive fantasies, and for the toddler whose baby does not come after such a long waiting these fantasies must seem corroborated. So this may be a difficult period not only because of the internal problems the woman has to face but also in the relationships which form a normal part of her everyday life and, in particular, the intense and demanding relationships within the nuclear family, and of a child who is demanding and difficult.

The bereaved mother needs someone who will take time to listen attentively, who can wait and be still, and who can respond sympathetically without herself feeling threatened by the loss and by the

* Cullberg, 'Mental Reactions of Women to Perinatal Death.'

intense emotions through which the mourner is passing. She needs someone who is content to reflect, contain and focus on the subject of grief without embarrassment, and without succumbing to the urge to off-load responsibility by giving direct counselling. This is what it is to share in the 'grief work'.

Antenatal preparation at its most worthwhile educates and supports couples in coping with a life crisis. Sometimes that crisis is not what we expect it to be, and instead of the adjustment required when a healthy baby is born there are the other necessary adjustments to the reality of loss. When we train women for labour only, or even for labour and the normal anticipated postnatal experience, we are in danger of focusing on a process and drawing a blueprint for it, which for some women is not going to be like that at all. This is where a narrow didactic method of childbirth education puts those women most at risk who confront an abnormal crisis, and where the broad approach allows them to make use of insights gained during the pregnancy to respond appropriately to whatever challenge lies ahead of them.

As I was starting to write this chapter I received a letter from a man whose wife I had first met after she had had a miscarriage which they had both found extremely disturbing. I asked them if they would like an opportunity to come and talk about it, which they did. Then she became pregnant again, and I saw them both at about fifteen weeks, when we had discussed their feelings about this pregnancy. Now she had had a premature stillbirth.

Shortly before the delivery she had heard her baby's heartbeats on the fetal monitor and the memory of this was foremost in her mind. After the delivery she was moved to a postnatal ward where she could hear the babies crying and as she later told me: 'They cried and I didn't have one. Every time I heard a baby crying or saw a baby I wanted to feed it.' Yet something extraordinary had happened, and the experience of losing the child was not shattering in the way that the previous miscarriage was. John, the husband, wrote,

In many ways it was a good experience . . . although it was a far more serious thing than the first miscarriage, we seem to have been much less screwed up by it. . . . It was something you couldn't argue with and could only rise to. Sarah was quite marvellous and even had room to spare among the sadness to be full of wonder and actual pleasure at the power of her body's opening up. The emotions are there in plenty, of course, but nothing seems to have been crushed or twisted or driven into a corner. Sarah is physically and emotionally recovering very quickly and it seems true that she's feeling better, more firmly rooted somehow, than she had done before.

I wondered if John interpreted what was happening in their lives in terms which were satisfying for him, but less so for Sarah—whether perhaps this is the way he wanted to see things, and *had* to see them to be able to tolerate the suffering. I rang them and spoke to her. She explained how when at last she was convinced by the doctors that the baby must be dead she agreed to an oxytocin drip, and that contractions lasting four minutes or so followed each other with increasing strength. I listened, and she added:

I know this will sound strange, but John and I felt it a marvellous experience. I was so fascinated and moved by my body taking over completely. I was amazed. The bearing down was marvellous too. There was nothing I need do because my body did the work.

And then she said, 'In the same way as teaching us not to fight the contractions, it could be that you've helped us not to fight the idea of losing the baby.'

Perhaps it is not only a question of helping people to meet the obvious crisis they are encountering at the moment but also of facilitating a flexible response to stress which can help them meet other life challenges of which they, and we, know nothing yet.

Bibliography

Argyle, Michael. *The Psychology of Interpersonal Behaviour*, London, Penguin, 1967.

Back, Kurt. *Beyond Words: The Story of Sensitivity Training and the Encounter Movement*, New York, Russell Sage Foundation, 1972.

Balint, Michael and Enid. *Psychotherapeutic Techniques in Medicine*, London, Tavistock Social Science Paperback, 1972.

Bax, Martin and Judy Bernal. *Your Child's First Five Years*, London, Heinemann, 1974.

Bean, Constance. *Methods of Childbirth*, New York, Doubleday, 1972.

Bing, Elizabeth. *Six Practical Lessons for an Easier Childbirth,* New York, Bantam Books, 1969.

Boston Women's Health Book Collective. *Our Bodies Ourselves*, 2nd edition, New York, Simon & Schuster, 1976.

Bourne, S. 'The Psychological Effects of Stillbirth on the Doctor', in N. Morris, ed., *Psychosomatic Medicine in Obstetrics and Gynaecology*, Basel, Karger, 1972.

Bradley, Robert A. *Husband-Coached Childbirth*, New York, Harper and Row, 1965.

Breen, Dana. *The Birth of a First Child*, London, Tavistock, 1975.

Buxton, R. St J. 'Maternal Respiration in Labour', London, *I.A.C.P.*, 1968.

Caldeyro-Barcia, R. 'Factors Controlling the Action of the Pregnant Human Uterus', in M. Knowlessor, ed., *Fifth Conference on*

Physiology of Prematurity, New York, Josiah Macey Jr. Foundation, 1961.

Caplan, G. *Principles of Preventive Psychiatry*, New York, Basic Books, 1964.

Chabon, Irving, *Awake and Aware*, New York, Dell Pub. Co., 1969.

Chamberlain Roma, et al. *British Births 1970*, London, Heinemann, 1975.

Colman, Arthur D. and Libby J. *Pregnancy: The Psychological Experience*, New York, Herder and Herder, 1972.

Csapo, A. 'The Mechanism of Myometrial Function and Its Disorders', in K. Bowes, ed., *Modern Trends in Obstetrics and Gynecology*, London, Butterworth, 1955.

Cullberg, J. 'Mental Reactions of Women to Perinatal Death', in N. Morris, ed., *Psychosomatic Medicine in Obstetrics and Gynaecology*, Basel, Karger, 1972.

Deutsch, Helene. *The Psychology of Women*, New York, Grune and Stratton, 1945.

Dickinson-Belskie. *Birth Atlas*, New York, Maternity Center Association.

Donnelly, Elizabeth. 'The Real of Her', *J. of Obstetrics, Gynecologic and Neonatal Nursing*, Vol. III, No. 3 (May/June), 1974.

Douglas, Mary. *Purity and Danger*, London, Penguin, 1970.

Downing, George, *The Massage Book*, London, Wildwood House Ltd., 1973.

Dunbar, Flanders. *Emotions and Bodily Changes*, New York, Columbia University Press, 1946.

Elenow, Allen J. and Scott N. Swischer, *Interviewing and Patient Care*, New York, O.U.P., 1972.

Evans-Pritchard, E. E. *Witchcraft, Oracles and Magic among the Azande*, London, O.U.P., 1937.

Ewy, Donna and Roger, eds., *Preparation for Childbirth*, Boulder, Colo., Pruett Pub. Co., 1970.

Fenn, Wallace O. and Hermann Rahn, eds., *Handbook of Physiology, Section 3, Respiration, Vol. I*, Washington, D.C., American Physiological Society, 1965.

Fisher, Seymour, and Sidney E. Cleveland, *Body Image and Personality*, New York, Dover Publications, 1968.

Flanagan, Geraldine Lux. *The First Nine Months of Life*, London, Heinemann, 1863.

Foulkes, S. H. and E. J. Anthony, *Group Psychotherapy*, London, Penguin, 1965.

Friedman, Emanual A. *Labor: Clinical Evaluation and Management*, New York, Appleton-Century-Crofts, 1967.

Garrey, M. M., et al., *Obstetrics Illustrated*, Edinburgh, Livingstone, 1969.

Goffman, Erving. *Interaction Ritual*, New York, Anchor, 1967.

——*The Presentation of Self in Everyday Life*, New York, Anchor, 1959.

Goldthorp, W. O., W. Hallam and J. Richman, 'Medical Knowledge in Gynaecological Patients – A Study of the Patient's Understanding of her Illness and Treatment', *Br. J. of Sexual Medicine*, 1975.

Gunther, Bernard. *Sense Relaxation Below Your Mind*, London, Macdonald, 1969.

Haire, Doris and John. *Implementing Family-Centred Maternity Care with a Central Nursery*, 3rd ed., Hillside. N.J., I.C.E.A., 1971.

Hazell, Lester D. *Commonsense Childbirth*, New York, G. P. Putnam's Sons, 1969.

Hollander M. H. and Thomas Szasz, *The Psychology of Medical Practice*, Philadelphia, Saunders, 1958.

Horney, Karen. *New Ways in Psychoanalysis*, 4th ed., London, Routledge, 1961.

Howard, A. 'The Hot-Cold Theory of Disease', *J. of Am. Med. Ass.*, Vol. 216, 1971.

Kitzinger, Sheila. *The Experience of Childbirth*, London, Gollancz 1962, Penguin 1967; New York, Taplinger 1972, Penguin, 1972.

——*Giving Birth—The Parents' Emotions in Childbirth*, England, Gollancz, 1971, Sphere, 1972; New York, Taplinger, 1972.

——*The Place of Birth*, edited by Sheila Kitzinger and Professor John Davis, and chapter 'Women's Experiences of Birth at Home', London, O.U.P., 1977.

——'Pregnancy—Time of Opportunity in Marriage' in *Marriage Guidance*, Vol. 12, 3, London, National Marriage Guidance Council, May, 1970.

——'The Woman on the Delivery Table' in *Woman on Woman*, edited by Margaret Laing, London, Sidgwick and Jackson, 1971.

——'Body Fantasies' in *New Society*, Vol. 21, 510, July 6, 1972.

——'West Indian Immigrant Children with Problems' in *Therapeutic Education*, edited by Giles, Jones and Wills, 1972.

——'An Anthropological Approach to Education for Childbirth with the Underprivileged' in *Psychosomatic Medicine in Obstetrics and Gynaecology*, edited by Norman Morris, Basel, Karger, 1972.

——'Speaking the Same Language', in *The Practitioner*, December, 1974.

——'Having a Baby in South Africa' in *The Third World*, London, New Society, 1976.

——'Touch Relaxation' in *The Family*, edited by Professor Herman Hirsch, Basel, Karger, 1976.

——'Image and Body Fantasy in Preparation for Birth? An Anthropological View' in *The Family*, edited by Professor Herman Hirsch, Basel, Karger, 1976.

——'Brief Encounters' in *The Practitioner*, August, 1976.

——'Journey Through Birth' (a set of cassette tape recordings), Julian Aston Productions, London and New York, 1976.

Klein, Melanie. *Love, Hate and Reparation*, London, Hogarth, 1953.

Lévi-Strauss, Claude. *Structural Anthropology*, New York, Anchor Books, 1967.

Lewis, A. E. 'Reactions to Stillbirth' in N. Morris, ed., *Psychosomatic Medicine in Obstetrics and Gynaecology*, Basel, Karger, 1972.

Llewelyn-Jones, Derek. *Fundamentals of Obstetrics & Gynaecology, Vol. I, Obstetrics*, London, Faber, 1973.

Lomas, Peter. 'The Significance of Post-Partum Breakdown' in *The Predicament of the Family*, London, Hogarth Press, 1972.

Lopata, Helena. *Occupation: Housewife*, New York, O.U.P. paperback, 1972.

Lumley J. et al., 'Hyperventilation in Obstetrics', *Am. J. Obstet. Gynec.*, March, 1969.

Macfarlane, Aidan. 'If a Smile Is So Important', *New Scientist*, April 25, 1974.

Masters, William, and Virginia Johnson, *Human Sexual Response*, Boston, Little, Brown, 1966.

——*Human Sexual Inadequacy*, Boston, Little, Brown, 1970.

Materozzo et al. *Psychotherapy*, Vol. 1, No. 3, 1965.

Melzack, Ronald. *The Puzzle of Pain*, London, Penguin, 1973.

Melzer, David. *Birth*, New York, Ballantine Books, 1973.

Miller, Jean Baker, ed., *Psychoanalysis and Women*, Baltimore, Penguin, 1973.

Montgomery, Eileen. *At Your Best for Birth and Later*, Bristol, John Wright, 1969.

Montagu, Ashley, *Touching: The Human Significance of the Skin*, New York, Columbia University Press, 1971.

Motoyama Etsuro K., et al. 'Adverse effect of Maternal Hyperventilation on the Foetus', *The Lancet*, February 5, 1966.

Newton, Niles. *The Family Book of Child Care*, New York, Harper and Row, 1957.

——*Maternal Emotions*, Jackson, Mississippi, Phronia Craft, 1958.

——'Interrelationships between Sexual Responsiveness, Birth and Breast Feeding', in Joseph Zubin and John Money, *Contemporary Sexual Behavior*, Baltimore, John Hopkins University Press, 1973.

New York Maternity Center, *A Baby is Born*, London, Allen & Unwin, 1966.

Nillson, Lennart, Axel Ingelman-Sundberg, Claes Wirsen, *The Everyday Miracle*, London, Penguin, 1967.

Oxorn, Harry, and William R. Foote. *Human Labor and Birth*, 2nd ed. London, Butterworths; New York, Appleton-Century-Crofts, 1968.

Painter, Charlotte. *Who Made the Lamb: the Intimate Journal of a Woman's Pregnancy and Childbirth* New York, Signet, 1966.

Parkes, Murray Colin. 'Grief as an Illness', *New Society*, April 1964.

——'Effects of Bereavement on Physical and Mental Health – A Study of the Medical Records of Widows', *Br. Med. J.* 2:274, 1964.

Randolph, Vance. *Ozark Superstitions*, New York, Columbia University Press, 1947.

Reeves, Jr., Robert B. 'The Hospital Chaplain Looks at Grief', in Bernard Schoenberg and others, *Loss and Grief: Psychological*

Management in Medical Practice, New York, Columbia University Press, 1970.

Richards, Martin. 'The One-day-old Deprived Child', *New Scientist*, March 28, 1974.

Richardson, Stephen and Alan Guttmacher, eds., *Social and Psychological Aspects of Childbearing*, Baltimore, Williams and Wilkins Co., 1967.

Roche, Peter. 'Somewhere on the Way', *The New Love Poetry*, London, Corgi, 1973.

Rombandeeva, E. I. 'Some Observances and Customs of the Mansi (Voguls) in Connection with Childbirth', V. Dioszeg, ed., *Popular Beliefs and Folklore Traditions in Siberia*, Bloomington, Indiana University Press, 1960.

Rush, Anne Kent. *Getting Clear: Body Work for Women*, London, Wildwood House, 1974.

Saling, E. 'The Effect on the Foetus of Maternal Hyperventilation during Labour', *J. Obstet. Gynaec. Br. Emp.*, Vol. 76, October 1969.

Schaffer, Rudolph. 'Behavioural Synchrony in Infancy', *New Society*, April 4, 1974.

Scully, Diana and Pauline Bart, 'A Funny Thing Happened on the Way to the Orifice', in Joan Huber, ed., *Changing Women in a Changing Society*, Chicago, University of Chicago Press, 1973.

Shearer, Madeleine. 'A Survey of the Literature on Ventilation and Hyperventilation in Childbirth', *Childbirth Education, Vol. II No. 4*, American Society for Psychoprophylaxis in Obstetrics, 1969.

Susser M. W. and W. Watson, *Sociology in Medicine*, 2nd Ed., London, O.U.P., 1971.

Tanzer, Deborah and Jean Block, *Why Natural Childbirth*, New York, Doubleday, 1972,

Velvovsky, I., K. Platonov, V. Ploticher and E. Schugom, *Painless Childbirth through Psychoprophylaxis*, Moscow, Foreign Languages Publishing House, 1960.

Wilson, John A., translator; James B. Pritchard, ed., *Ancient Near Eastern Texts Relating to the Old Testament*, 2nd ed., Princeton, N.J., Princeton University Press, 1955.

Williams, Margaret. *Keeping Fit for Pregnancy and Labour*, London, National Childbirth Trust, 1969.

——and Dorothy Booth. *Antenatal Education: Guidelines for Teachers*, Edinburgh, Churchill Livingstone, 1974.

Winnicott, D. W. *The Maturational Processes and the Facilitating Environment*, New York, International Universities Press, 1965.

Zweig, Stefan. *In Quest of Fellowship*, London, Heinemann, 1965.

Index

Index